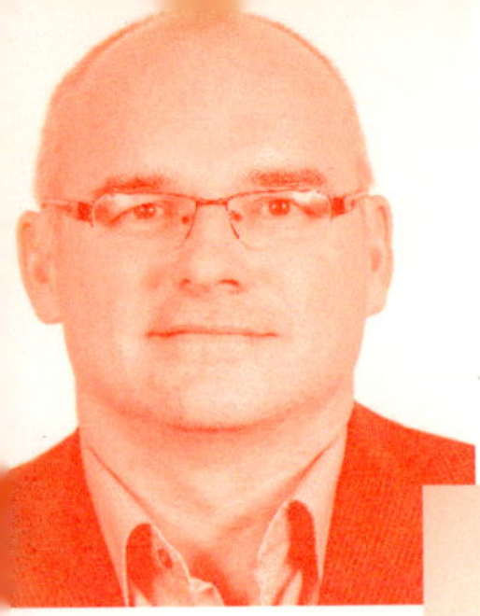
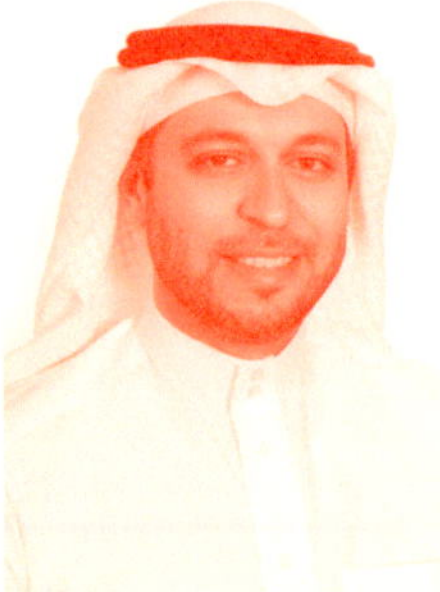
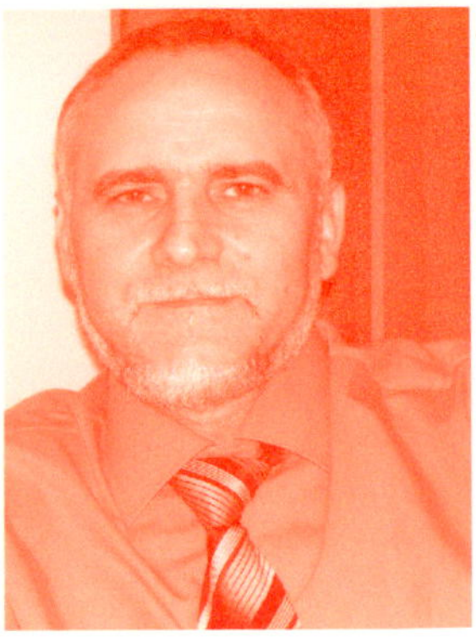
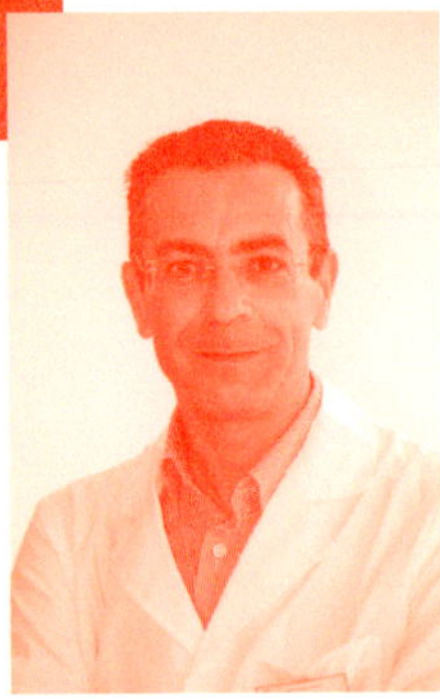
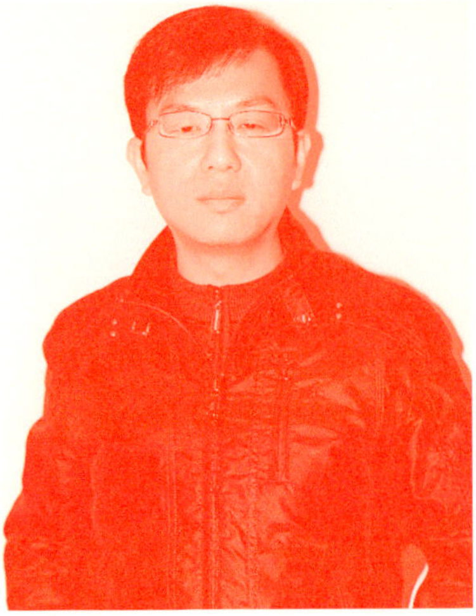
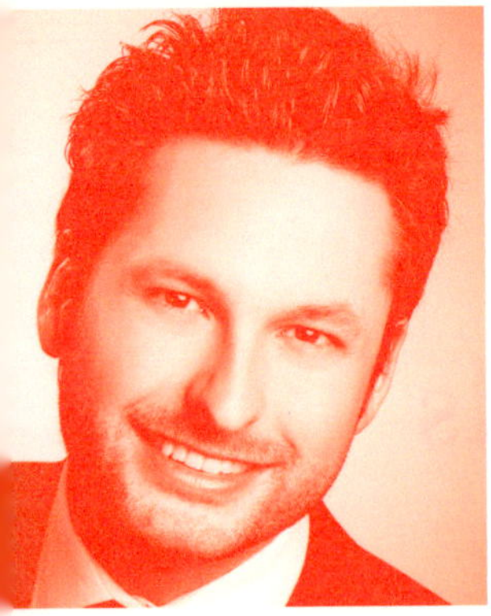
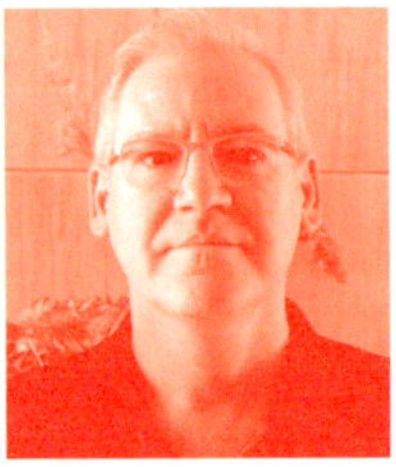

IntechOpen

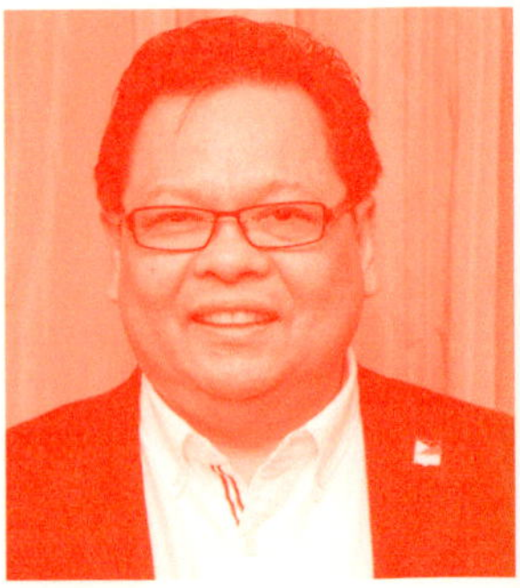
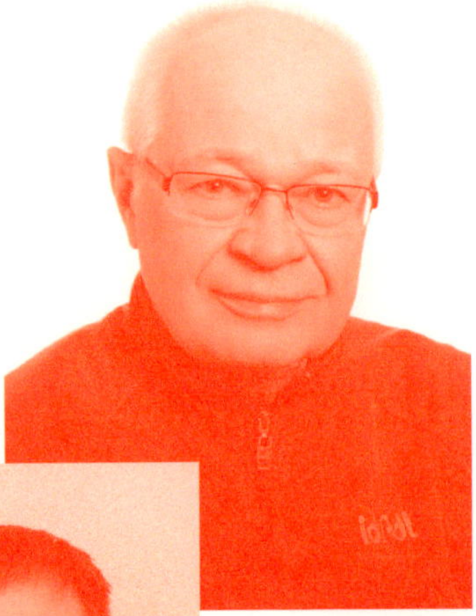
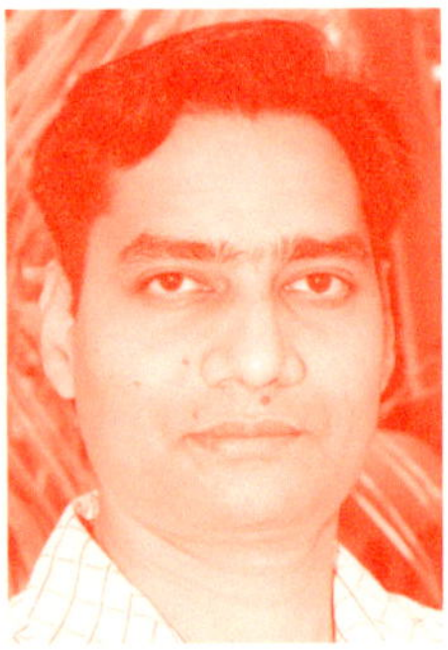
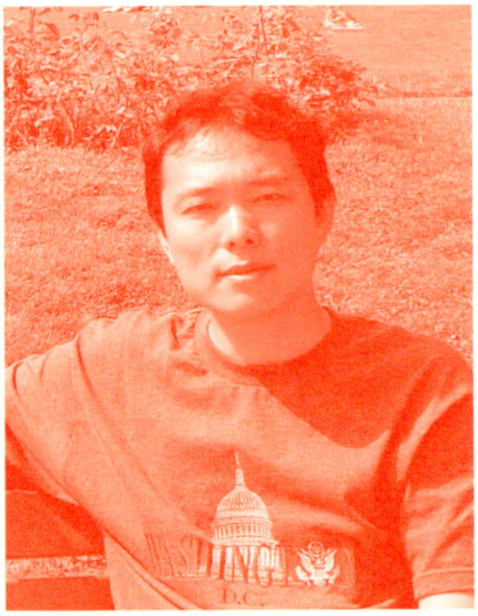
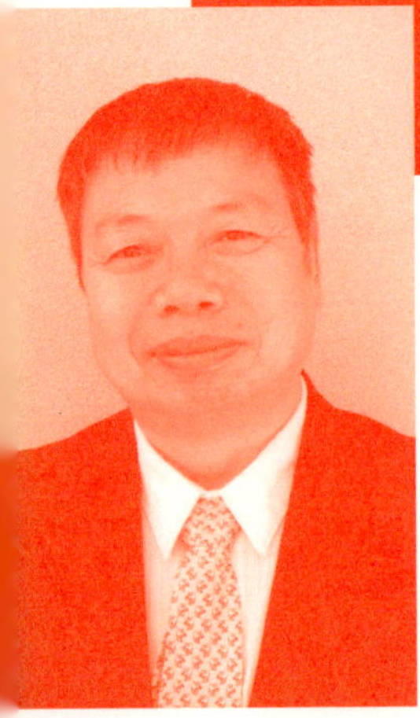
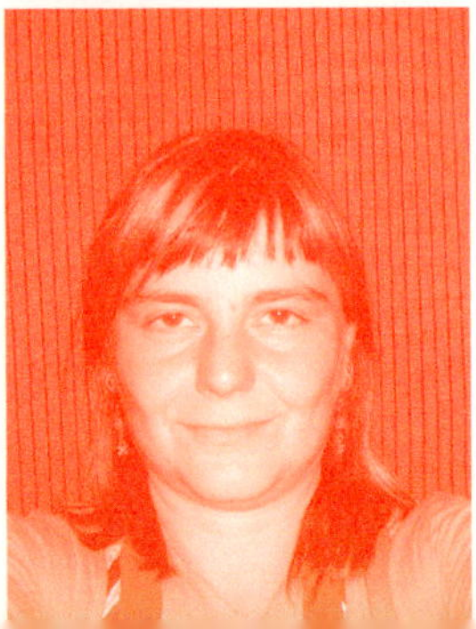

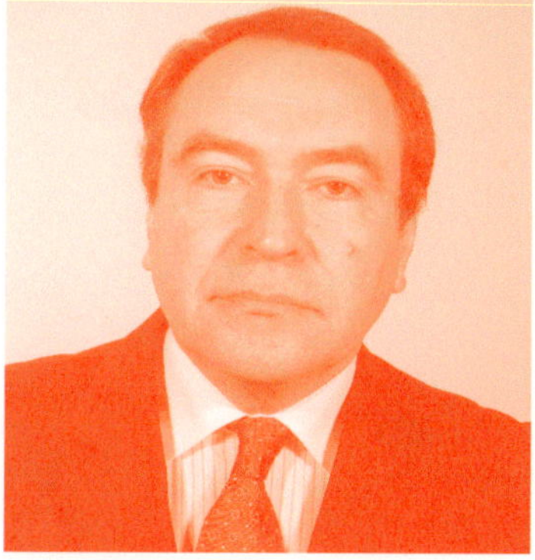

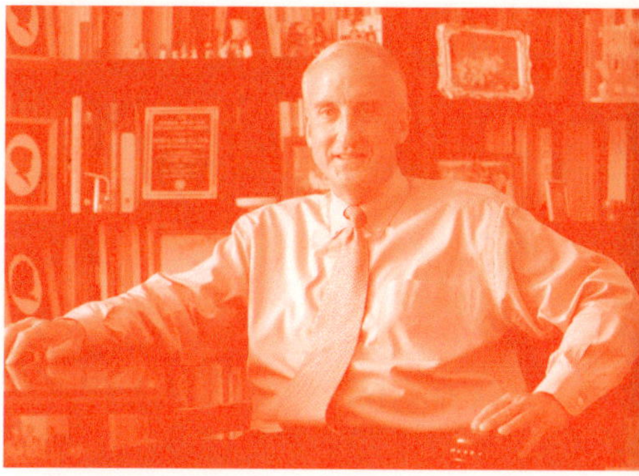

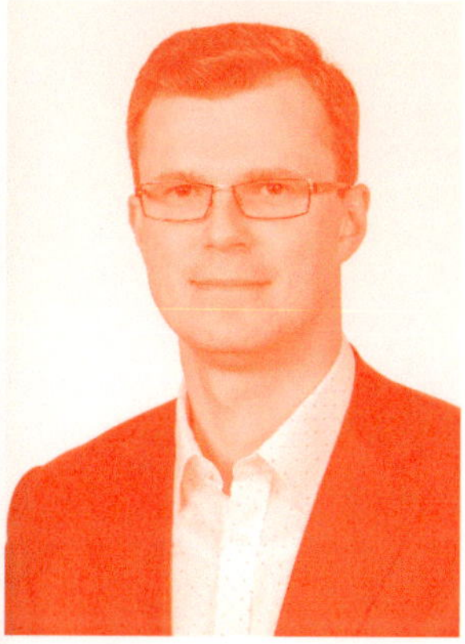

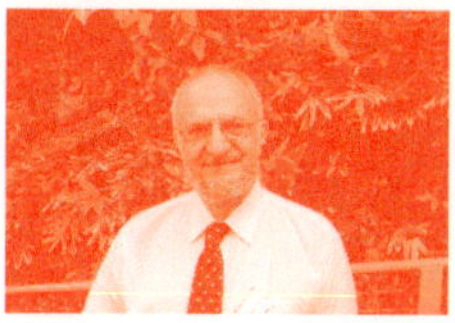

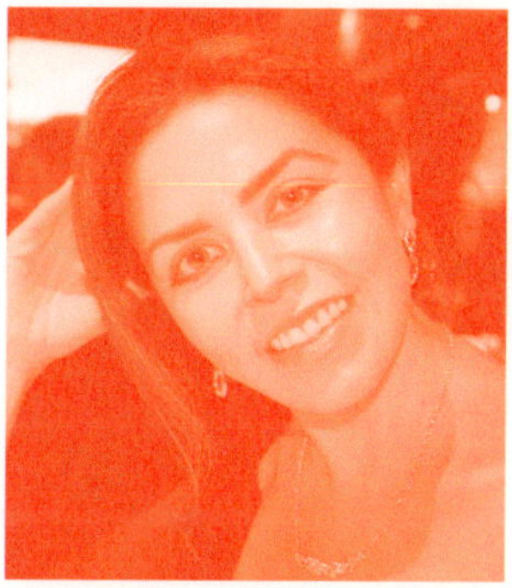

Supporting open minds since 2005

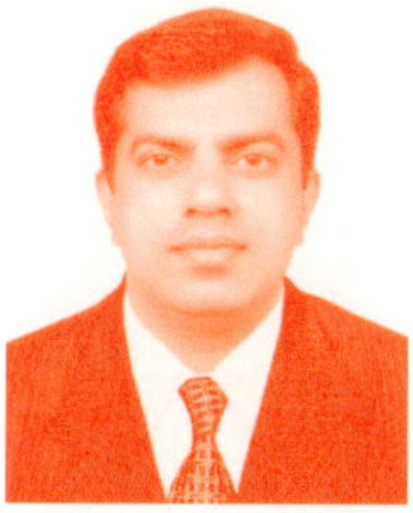

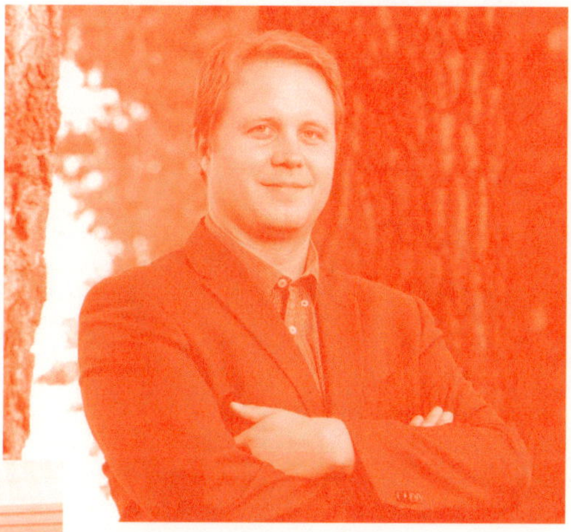

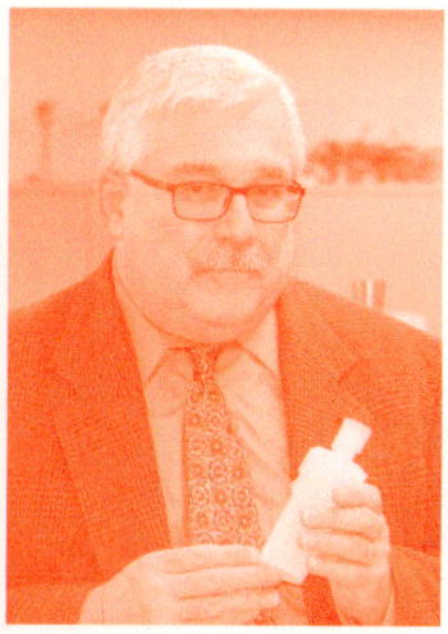

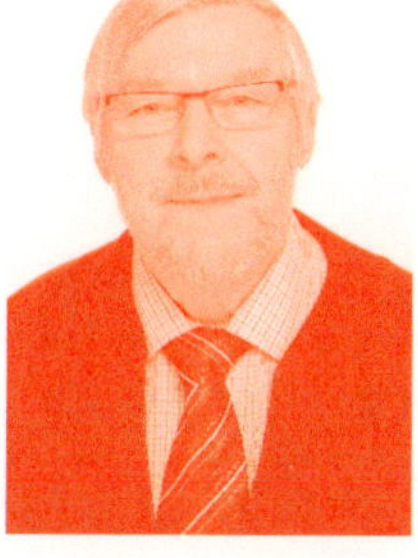

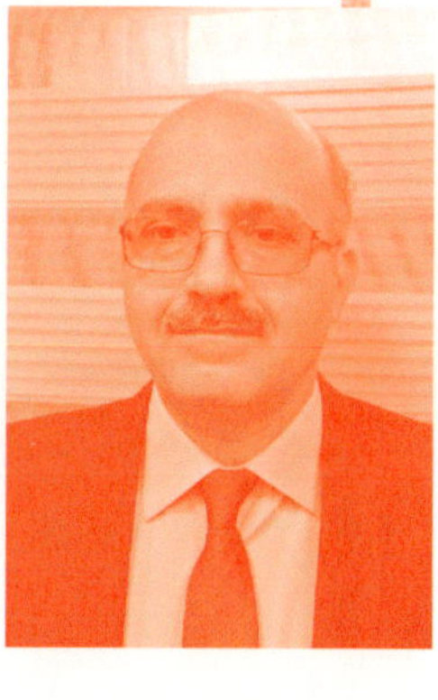

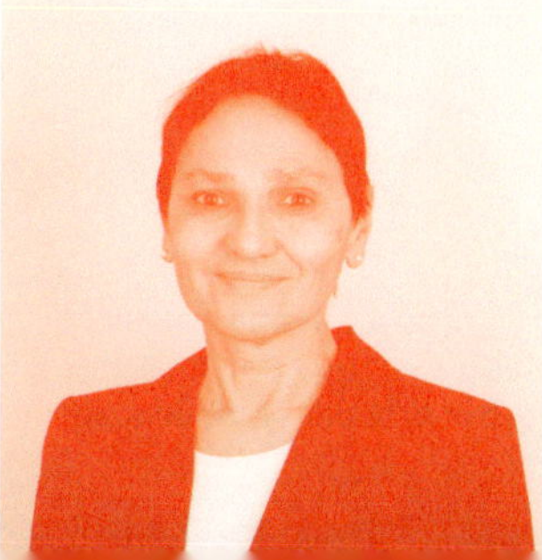

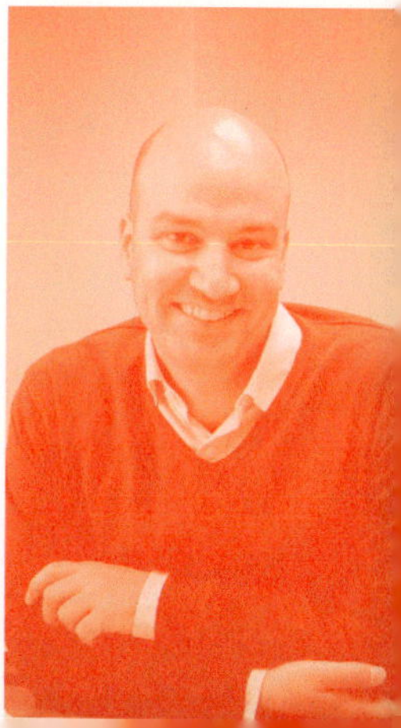

Novel Diagnostic Methods in Ophthalmology
http://dx.doi.org/10.5772/intechopen.79334
Edited by Anna Nowinska

Part of IntechOpen Book Series: Biomedical Engineering, Volume 6
Book Series Editor: Robert Koprowski

Contributors
Chao-Min Cheng, Yu-Ting Tsao, Wei-Hsuan Sung, Hung-Chi Chen, Min-Yen Hsu, Samet Gulkas, Osman Cekic, Seyhan Topbas, Nazmiye Erol, Mustafa Deger Bilgec, Jesus Hernan Gonzalez-Cortes, Abraham Olvera-Barrios, Jesus Mohamed-Hamsho, Jesus Emiliano Gonzalez-Cantu, Silvia Tavazzi, Alessandra Parodi, Sara Colciago, Gabriele Nigrotti, Simone Borghesi, Fabrizio Zeri, Robin Ross, Jason Singh, Mandi Conway, Gholam Peyman, Sami Kabbara, Robin Demi Ross, David Rosen, Leonardo Montilla, Charles Ingram

First published in London, United Kingdom, 2019 by IntechOpen
IntechOpen is the global imprint of INTECHOPEN LIMITED, registered in England and Wales, registration number: 11086078, The Shard, 25th floor, 32 London Bridge Street
London, SE19SG – United Kingdom
Printed in Croatia

British Library Cataloguing-in-Publication Data
A catalogue record for this book is available from the British Library

Additional hard and PDF copies can be obtained from orders@intechopen.com

Novel Diagnostic Methods in Ophthalmology
Edited by Anna Nowinska
p. cm.
Print ISBN 978-1-83880-311-7
Online ISBN 978-1-83880-312-4
eBook (PDF) ISBN 978-1-83881-853-1
ISSN 2631-5343

For EU product safety concerns:
IN TECH d.o.o., Prolaz Marije Krucifikse Kozulić 3, 51000 Rijeka, Croatia, info@intechopen.com or visit our website at intechopen.com.

IntechOpen Book Series
Biomedical Engineering
Volume 6

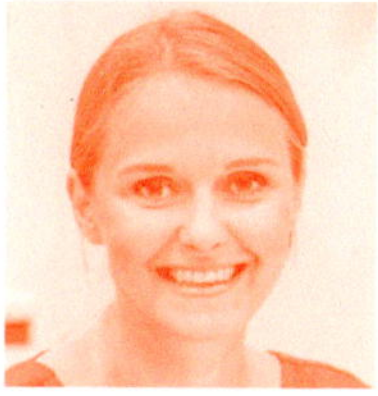

Dr. Anna Karolina Nowinska habilitated doctor of ophthalmology, adjunct at Chair and Department of Ophthalmology; School of Medicine with the Division of Dentistry in Zabrze, Medical University of Silesia in Katowice (Poland). Dr. Nowinska is a member of the Polish Society of Ophthalmology and the Association for Research in Vision and Ophthalmology. Her areas of scientific expertise include corneal dystrophies and degenerations, and anterior and posterior eye segment optical coherence tomography. She is the author of over 30 original articles, 5 monographs, and over 100 abstracts presented during international and Polish meetings. Dr. Nowinska also has over 10 years' experience in ophthalmic surgery, with special interest in cataract and vitreoretinal surgery.

Editor of Volume 6:
Anna Nowinska
Chair and Department of Ophthalmology, School of Medicine with the Division of Dentistry in Zabrze, Medical University of Silesia, Katowice, Poland

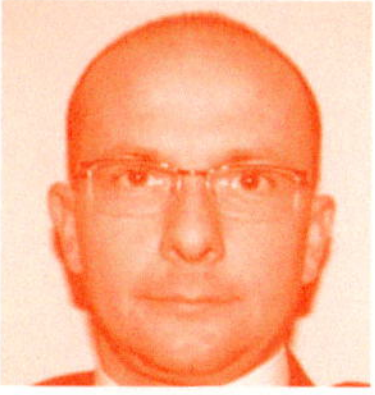

Robert Koprowski, MD (1997), PhD (2003), Habilitation (2015), is a lecturer at the Department of Biomedical Computer Systems, Institute of Computer Science, University of Silesia, Poland. For 20 years, he has been dealing with analysis and processing of biomedical images with a particular emphasis on the full automation of measurement for a large inter-individual variability of patients. He is the author of dozens of papers with an impact factor (IF) and more than a hundred of other papers as well as the author or coauthor of six books. Additionally, he is the author of several national and international patents in the field of biomedical devices and imaging. Since 2011, he has been a reviewer of grants and projects (including EU projects) in the field of biomedical engineering.

Book Series Editor:
Robert Koprowski
University of Silesia, Poland

Scope of the Series

Biomedical engineering is one of the fastest growing interdisciplinary branches of science and industry. The combination of electronics and computer science with biology and medicine has resulted in improved patient diagnosis, reduced rehabilitation time and better quality of life. Nowadays, all medical imaging devices, medical instruments or new laboratory techniques are the result of the cooperation of specialists in various fields. The series of biomedical engineering books covers such areas of knowledge as chemistry, physics, electronics, medicine and biology. This series is intended for doctors, engineers and scientists involved in biomedical engineering or those wanting to start working in this field.

Contents

Preface

This book intends to provide the reader with a comprehensive overview of the current and novel ocular diagnostic methods of the anterior and posterior eye segment used in clinical practice as well as in scientific projects. It is intended to interest both clinical ophthalmologists and researchers interested in projects involving ocular imaging.

The chapters include the theoretical basis as well as practical approach and usage of the following techniques: endothelial microscopy and corneal pachymetry, optical coherence tomography, endoOCT, wide-field retinal imaging, ultrasound imaging, and innovative diagnostic tools for ophthalmology in low-income countries.

The book sections are created according to ocular compartments: anterior and posterior eye segment.

Silvia Tavazzi et al. describe the novel approach of analyzing the cornea and morphology and morphometry of corneal endothelium with a slit lamp equipped with a high-resolution digital sensor. This innovative approach allows rapid diagnosis of corneal endothelial dystrophies and other endothelial abnormalities.

Yu-Ting Tsao et al. introduce a promising approach of a paper-based ELISA method to assess vascular endothelial growth factor level in aqueous humor, which could be an important indicator in diseases such as uveitis, diabetic retinopathy, and age-related macular degeneration. The possible potential of this method may interest researchers and could also become a diagnostic test in clinical practice.

A few chapters are devoted to recently introduced wide-field retinal imaging and intraoperative optical coherence tomography. The authors present the technical background of the methods, commercially available devices, as well as many clinical examples of intraoperative usage in vitreoretinal surgery, especially in macular surgery in diseases such as epiretinal membranes, macular holes, and vitreoretinal traction syndrome.

Jason Singh et al. focus on an emerging issue of ocular examination in low-income countries describing available low-cost diagnostic methods and resources that aim to assist in the fight against preventable blindness, such as smartphone-integrated fundoscopy, laptop size ocular ultrasonography, or self-adjustable glasses.

To conclude, the book intends to provide valuable information in terms of anterior and posterior eye segment diagnostic methods, which could be used in everyday clinical practice to allow early diagnosis of diseases such as corneal dystrophies, keratoconus, cataract, central and peripheral retinal disorders, and optic neuropathies.

It also provides a very detailed description of the novel intraoperative technique of optical coherence tomography, which is very promising in improving the quality of vitreoretinal surgery.

Anna Nowinska
Chair and Department of Ophthalmology,
School of Medicine with the Division of Dentistry in Zabrze,
Medical University of Silesia,
Katowice, Poland

Section 1

Anterior Eye Segment Diagnostic Methods

Chapter 1

Corneal Pachymetry and Endothelial Microscopy by Slit-Lamp

Silvia Tavazzi, Alessandra Parodi, Sara Colciago, Gabriele Nigrotti, Simone Borghesi and Fabrizio Zeri

Abstract

A slit-lamp biomicroscope Visionix VX75 has been equipped with a high-resolution digital sensor. A specular reflection technique at an angular magnification of 36× performed by the slit-lamp biomicroscope is used to develop a procedure to (i) measure the thickness of the human cornea by measuring the distance between the two reflections of its anterior and posterior surfaces and (ii) capture suitable images for morphometric analyses of the corneal endothelium's cell mosaic. The examples of morphometric analysis of these images are reported. The biases due to the dioptric power of the anterior surface of the cornea, the oblique observation, and the asymmetry of the digital biomicroscope are discussed. These biases can be corrected by a specific calibration.

Keywords: slit-lamp biomicroscope, pachymetry, endothelial microscopy, specular reflection, morphometric analysis

1. Introduction

The slit-lamp biomicroscope is an instrument widely used by ophthalmologists and optometrists to observe the anterior segment of the eye. The instrument is composed by two main components: an illumination system, the slit-lamp, and an observation system, the biomicroscope. They can be set up in different configurations allowing several types of illumination techniques. One of these is the specular reflection: the examiner directs the incident light toward the eye with angle of incidence α on the anterior surface of the cornea, then sets the angle between the illumination system and the biomicroscope at 2α, and observes the bright reflection on the anterior surface through the biomicroscope. Usually the angle 2α is relatively high, ranging from 40 to 70°. The intense reflection is due to the change of refractive index between the air and the anterior surface of the cornea. A digital camera coupled with the right or left eyepiece tube can be used to capture images. Part of the light reaching the observation system is deviated by a beam splitter toward a converging lens, which allows the formation of a real image on the plane of the digital sensor.

The configuration of the specular reflection can also be used to observe the reflection from the posterior surface of the cornea (endothelium) due to the change of refractive index between the corneal endothelium and aqueous humor. However, this second reflection is much less evident than the previous one because of the smaller variation of refractive index between the two adjacent components. To observe the posterior reflection, light coming from the illumination system is focalized on the posterior surface and generates an image of the illuminated slit. The correct focus may be reached through the eyepieces' view, and a real image is detected on the digital sensor. In this configuration, only the posterior corneal surface (within the depth of field of the system) is in focus. This surface is optically conjugated with the plane of the sensor. A sort of slit image is also formed on the anterior surface of the cornea, but it is not a perfectly focused image of the slit and, consequently, neither is the resulting image on the sensor of the biomicroscope.

When a relatively narrow slit is used, the distance on the sensor between the in-focus image and the other image of the slit (formed by reflected beams from posterior and anterior surfaces, respectively) can be used to deduce the thickness of the cornea (pachymetry). A relatively narrow beam is recommended to reduce uncertainty in finding the distance between the two surfaces, i.e., the corneal thickness. Corneal pachymetry is a technique used in clinical practice for monitoring different conditions such as the progress of corneal diseases, to evaluate suitable patients before refractive surgery, and to determine intraocular pressure. During routine examination by slit-lamp biomicroscope, corneal thickness can also be measured by considering the apparent thickness of the optical section of the cornea [1]. Other methods are ultrasound pachymetry, optical coherence tomography, Scheimpflug imaging [2–15].

With a larger slit, the endothelium cell mosaic can be seen adjacent to the region of the intense light reflection from the anterior surface. The corneal endothelium is a cell monolayer laying on the posterior surface of the cornea. It regulates the transport of solutes and water across the interface between the cornea and anterior chamber of the eye. Pathologies such as the narrow-angle glaucoma, iritis, and corneal dystrophies can change the shape and size of the endothelial cells and their number per unit area, as well as trauma, aging, intraocular surgery, drugs, and wear of contact lenses [16–20]. A significant loss of cells is typically accompanied by an increase in the variability of cell size (polymegethism) and shape (polymorphism). Endothelium analysis is often carried out by automatic instruments, while the analysis by a digital slit-lamp biomicroscope is less expensive and allows to observe any specific region of interest of the cornea, so that a more complete characterization of the endothelium can be achieved. However, the common cell recognition methods are often not applicable to images taken by a slit-lamp biomicroscope. The main problem is typically the lack of information in some parts of the cells' borders [21]. A recent method was reported in 2016 allowing an improved cell recognition and morphometric analysis [22]. It was applied to a Takagi 700 GL LED biomicroscope equipped with TD-10 digital camera.

This chapter describes the results obtained by a Visionix VX75 slit-lamp biomicroscope equipped with a high-resolution digital sensor. We captured in vivo images of the two reflections from anterior and posterior corneal surfaces to deduce corneal thickness (pachymetry). We took images of the corneal endothelium with larger slits. They show the typical cell mosaic, and they are suitable for morphometric analysis. The effects of the dioptric power of the anterior surface of the cornea, of the oblique observation, and of the asymmetry of the digital biomicroscope on morphometric analysis are also discussed. The effects of these potential systematic errors can be greatly reduced by a preliminary calibration.

2. Methods

A Visionix VX75 slit-lamp biomicroscope equipped with a digital sensor Matrix Vision (sensor size, 2464 × 2056 pixels; pixel size, 3.45 × 3.45 μm^2; maximum number of frames per second, 35) was used with an angular magnification setting of the biomicroscope equal to 36×. A dedicated software was developed to take images through this sensor. A live digital magnification controlled by the operator was also applied to facilitate image acquisition. Images of the illuminated slit on the posterior surface of human corneas were taken in vivo both in the case of relatively narrow slits (for pachymetry analyses) and in the case of larger slits (for endothelial microcopy analyses). A sequence of MATLAB functions was created for the analysis of the images.

3. Slit-lamp biomicroscope corneal pachymetry

Figure 1 shows an example of image of the two reflections from the anterior corneal surface (slit image not perfectly in focus) and from the posterior surface (slit image in focus) taken at 36× on the central portion of the cornea of a young adult.

General equations on the relationship between true corneal thickness t and apparent corneal thickness s observed by a biomicroscope at oblique observation are reported in the literature [23, 24]. These equations can also be applied to the specific configuration of specular reflection. In this case, s is the lateral distance between the two reflections from anterior and posterior corneal surfaces, such as those of **Figure 1**. **Figure 2** is inspired by a figure reported in Brennan et al. [23], from which the following Eqs. (1)–(3) are also deduced:

$$\frac{R}{t} \sim \frac{R}{s}(c_1 + c_2)\cos\phi_2 + \frac{k_1 + k_2}{c_1 + c_2} - \frac{1}{2}(c_1 - c_2)\tan(\phi_2) \tag{1}$$

where t is the true thickness, s is the apparent thickness (viz., the distance between the two reflections in the case of specular reflection), and R is the

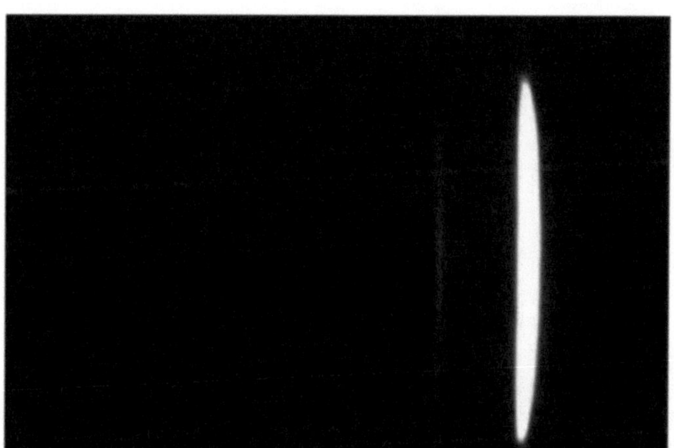

Figure 1.
Example of the two reflections from the anterior corneal surface (slit image on the right, not perfectly in focus) and from the posterior surface (slit image on the left, in focus) taken on the central portion of the cornea of a young adult by a Visionix VX75 slit-lamp biomicroscope at 36×.

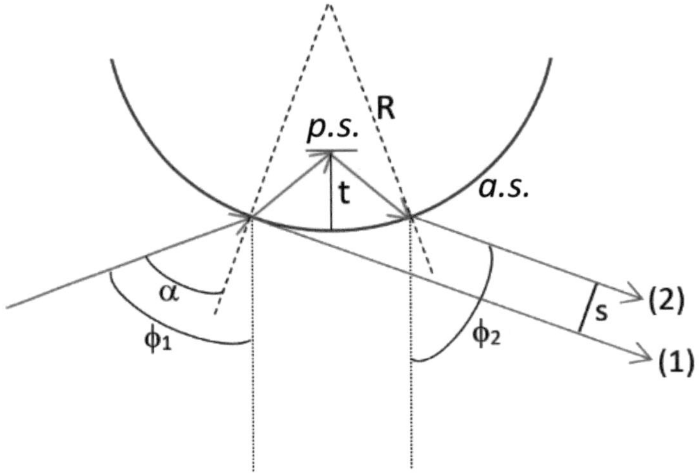

Figure 2.
Scheme showing apparent thickness s *and true thickness* t *of a sample (e.g., the human cornea) with spherical anterior surface (curvature radius R) as reported by Brennan et al. [23, 24].* ϕ_1 *and* ϕ_2 *are the angles that appear in Eqs. (1)–(3) [23]. Labels* p.s. *and* a.s. *indicate the posterior surface and the anterior surface, respectively. Labels (1) and (2) indicate the rays of light reflected from the anterior and posterior surfaces, respectively, in the configuration of specular reflection.*

curvature radius of the anterior surface. Angles ϕ_1 and ϕ_2 are shown in **Figure 2**; c_j and k_j are

$$c_j = \frac{1}{\sqrt{\frac{n^2}{\sin^2(\phi_j)} - 1}} \tag{2}$$

$$k_j = c_j + \frac{c_j^3}{2} - \frac{c_j^2 n^2}{\tan\left(\phi_j\right) \sin^2\left(\phi_j\right)} \tag{3}$$

where j = 1, 2 and n is the cornea refractive index (n = 1.376 [25]).

In the specific case of specular reflection, angles ϕ_1 and ϕ_2 are equal ($\phi_1 = \phi_2 = \phi$) and Eq. (1) can be written as

$$\frac{R}{t} \sim \frac{R}{s}\left(\frac{2}{\sqrt{\frac{n^2}{\sin^2(\phi)} - 1}}\right) cos\phi + 1 + \frac{1}{2\left[\frac{n^2}{\sin^2(\phi)} - 1\right]} - \frac{n^2}{\tan(\phi)\sin^2(\phi)\sqrt{\frac{n^2}{\sin^2(\phi)} - 1}} \tag{4}$$

In the limit case of a flat sample (R → ∞), Eq. (4) reduces to

$$t = \frac{s}{2\cos(\alpha)\tan\left(arcsin\left(\frac{sin(\alpha)}{n}\right)\right)} \tag{5}$$

By measuring the distance s between the two reflections observed in the image (e.g., as in **Figure 1**), from Eq. (4), we deduce the true corneal thickness t. However, this procedure contains a systematic error. The image of **Figure 1** was taken with an angular magnification setting of the biomicroscope equal to 36× and the angle between the axis of the illumination system, and the axis of the biomicroscope was fixed at 45°. Therefore, to a first approximation, the angle 2° can be set to be 45°. However, this assumption contains a systematic error due to the asymmetry of digital biomicroscopes [24]. Indeed, the sensor of a digital biomicroscope is positioned either at the right or at the left eyepiece of the biomicroscope (left side in the case of the Visionix VX75 biomicroscope). The sample is typically slightly rotated by an angle γ to direct the light beam into the correct channel of the biomicroscope and reach the sensor, as discussed in Ref. [24]. For the Visionix VX75 biomicroscope, γ was measured to be about 2.5°. During the acquisition of the image reported in **Figure 1**, the illumination system was positioned to the right of the examiner and the biomicroscope to the left. The digital sensor was placed on the left eyepiece of the biomicroscope, so that the true angle between the incident beam and the beam directed to the sensor is not the angle 2ϕ between illumination and biomicroscope, but it is equal to $2(\phi + \gamma)$. Therefore, due to this asymmetry of the digital biomicroscope, ϕ_1 and ϕ_2 in **Figure 2** and ϕ in Eq. (4) must be replaced with $(\phi + \gamma)$, i.e., about 25° in the considered case. Considering this aspect, the measure of s by the slit-lamp biomicroscope determines the thickness t. As discussed in Section 5, the bias in this procedure can be corrected by a system calibration.

4. Slit-lamp biomicroscope endothelial microscopy

Figure 3 shows few examples of images of the corneal endothelium of different subjects taken through the 36× objective. A different view of the corneal endothelium of a young adult is reported in **Figure 4**. The x and y coordinates corresponding to the image plane are shown on two axes. The third axis (z) shows the luminance of the image at each pixel.

Corneal endothelium can be described by endothelial cell density (ECD), cell hexagonality (HEX), and coefficient of variation (CoV). ECD is the number of cells per unit area. HEX is the percentage of cells with six nearest-neighbor cells, also defined as the percentage of six-sided cells. CoV is the ratio between standard deviation and mean value of the areas of the cells. As already mentioned, a significant loss of cells due to specific pathologies causes a decrease of ECD, and it is typically accompanied by an increase in the variability of cell size (polymegethism) and shape (polymorphism). However, the correlation between ECD and the other two parameters is typically poor because the measured ECD value (in contrast to HEX and CoV) depends on factors such as (i) the magnification of the images produced by the anterior surface of the cornea, which can vary from subject to subject, and (ii) the intrinsic cell size, which may also vary from subject to subject, even in the presence of perfectly regular hexagonal mosaics. On the contrary, a negative correlation is expected between CoV and HEX [26–30]: the higher the polymegethism (relatively high CoV), the higher the polymorphism (relatively low HEX).

ECD, HEX, and CoV can be deduced from images such as those reported in **Figures 3** and **4**. The computation of those parameters on a sample involves a lengthy counting process, if manually done by an operator. An automated way of determining such parameters is therefore desirable. The starting point is capturing a good quality image of the endothelium, inside which the operator can select a region of interest, preferably containing a few hundreds of cells (to get a statistically significant sample [31]) with sharp details uniformly illuminated. An automatized sequence of MATLAB functions acting on this region of interest was created. The purpose is, at first, to automatically detect cells' boundaries as accurately as possible and then to compute relevant cells' statistics from them. The following figures highlight some intermediate steps of the procedure. **Figure 5** shows the selection of the area of interest while **Figure 6** the obtained partition of the region of interest

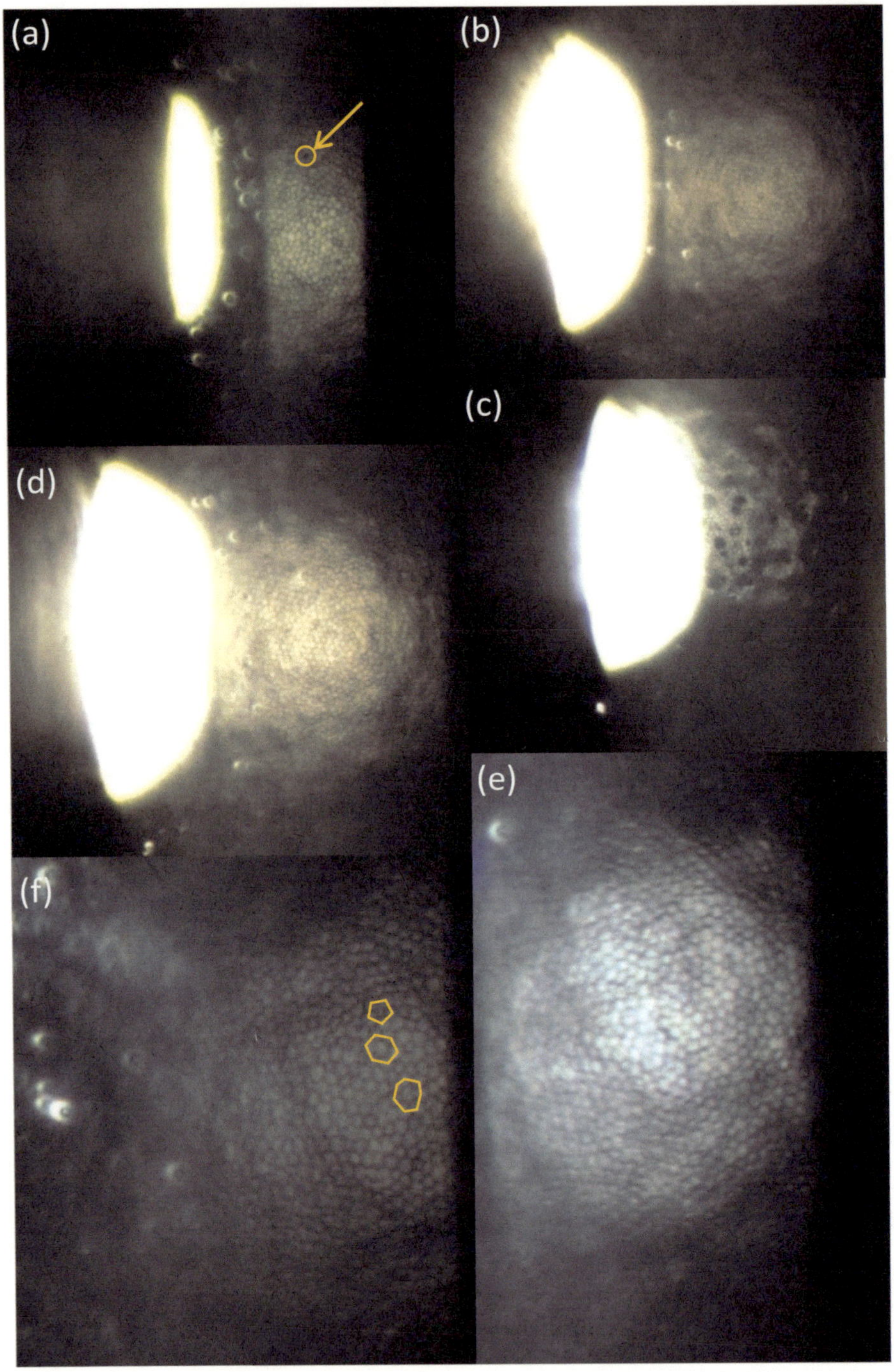

Figure 3.
Examples of images (a–d) and examples of enlarged portions of images (e, f) of the corneal endothelium of different subjects taken by a Visionix VX75 slit-lamp biomicroscope at 36×. In (a), a circle with an arrow indicates how a typical endothelial bleb appears. In (c), several endothelial guttae can be observed. In (f), a hexagon shows the typical hexagonal packing of regular mosaics of endothelial cells where each cell has six nearest neighbors. The other two closed polygons highlight 5 and 7 nearest-neighbor cells, respectively.

along cells' boundaries. Finally, in **Figure 7** we display the histograms of cells' area and the histograms of cells' gonality. The gonality of a cell is defined as the number of cells that are its nearest neighbors; sometimes it is also defined as the number of

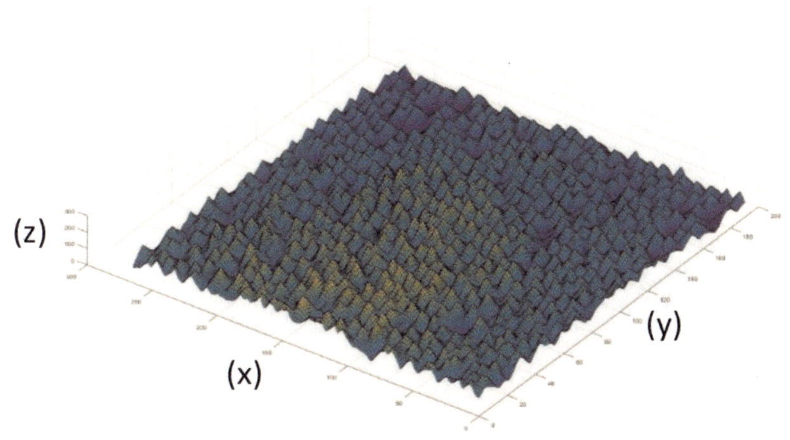

Figure 4.
View of a portion of the cell mosaic of the corneal endothelium of a young adult taken by a Visionix VX75 slit-lamp biomicroscope at 36×. The x and y coordinates corresponding to the image plane are shown on two axes. The third axis (z) shows the luminance of the image.

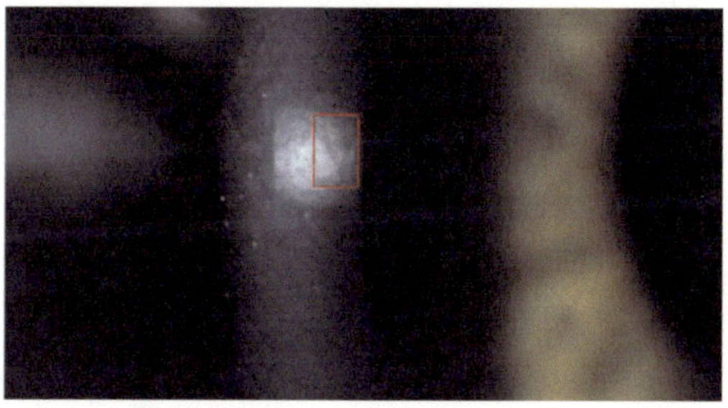

Figure 5.
Selection of the region of interest on the image of a corneal endothelium taken by slit-lamp biomicroscope.

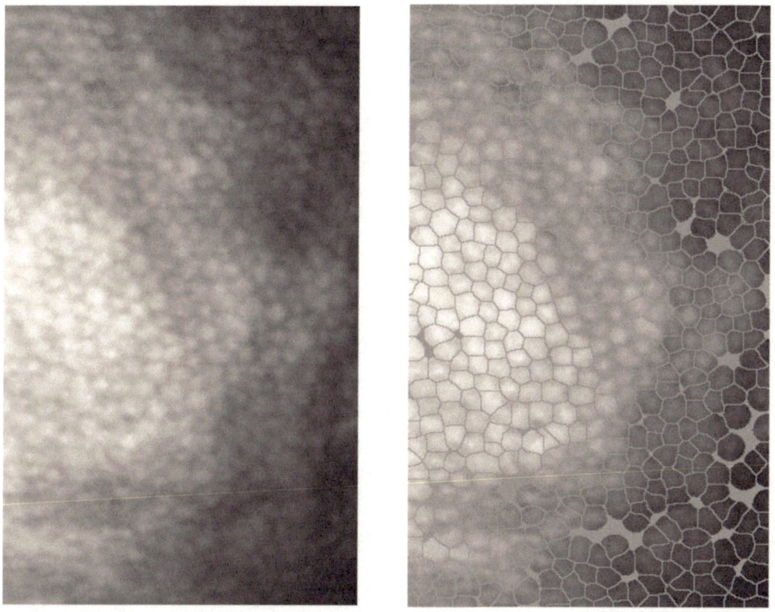

Figure 6.
Region of interest zoomed and partitioned along cells' boundaries.

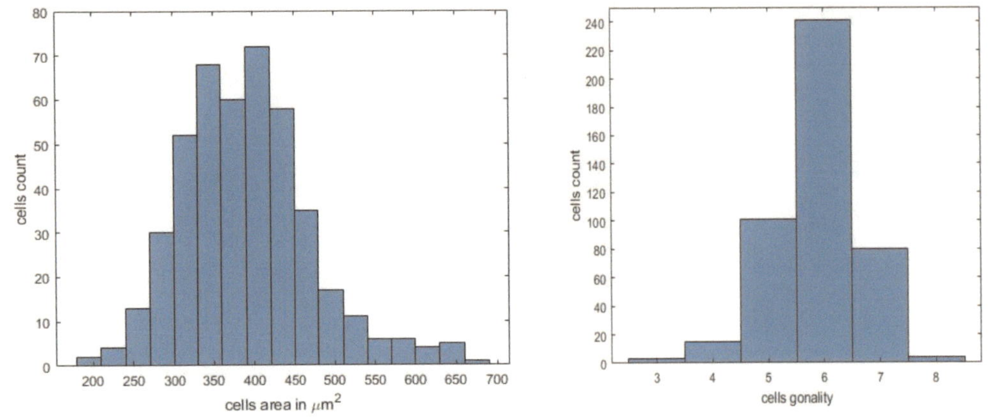

Figure 7.
Cells' area distribution (left) and cells' gonality distribution (right).

sides of the cell. In the specific example of **Figures 5–7**, MATLAB functions selected 444 cells for data computations.

A few aspects must be considered, for a quantitative evaluation of the parameters ECD, HEX, and CoV: firstly, the effects on ECD of the image magnification due to the dioptric power of the corneal anterior surface. ECD can be evaluated by the ratio N/A, where N is the number of recognized cells in a selected area A. The dioptric power of the corneal anterior surface induces a magnification on the sensor of this area, thus requiring the correction of the measured density to obtain the true value of ECD. In addition to the magnification produced by the anterior surface of the cornea, the angle of observation is another aspect that influences the area of the image [22]. The posterior corneal surface is indicated by a segment in **Figure 2** with label *p.s.* Its image is captured along the direction indicated by the ray (2) in the same figure. The larger the angle of observation, the larger the portion of internal surface projected onto the plane of the sensor. In other words, the cells in the image are narrowed along one direction. If not accounted for, this shrinkage is responsible for the increase of the measured cell density on the sensor due to the larger angle of observation. Moreover, the correction for such an angle presents the same issues discussed above, concerning the asymmetry of digital biomicroscopes. During the acquisition of the images reported in **Figures 3** and **4**, the illumination system was positioned on the left and the biomicroscope on the right. The digital sensor was on the left eyepiece of the biomicroscope, so that the true angle of the incident beam and the true angle of observation are not ϕ, but $(\phi - \gamma)$, i.e., about 20° in the considered case. As discussed in Section 5, a calibration with a suitable sample corrects these errors. Interestingly, the inaccuracy induced by the dioptric power of the anterior corneal surface, by the oblique observation, and by the asymmetry of the digital biomicroscope affects only ECD measurements. Unlike ECD, the other two parameters, HEX and CoV, are not influenced by the magnification factor because they are not influenced by possible errors in the measurement of the selected area A.

5. Reference standard sample for calibration

By what is discussed in the previous section, a calibration is recommended before a quantitative analysis of the corneal thickness (Section 3) and the endothelial cell density (Section 4). For this purpose, images of a planar reference grid should be taken at the desired angular magnification setting of the biomicroscope. The linear magnification of the real image on the sensor can be computed as the ratio between the size of the image of the elements of the reference grid and the size of the reference grid itself.

While the calibration through a planar grid can correct for errors induced by the lateral shrinkage of the image caused by the oblique observation and the biomicroscope's asymmetry, it will not account for issues related to the dioptric power of cornea's anterior surface. One further calibration employing a reference lens, such as the standard samples proposed in Refs. [22, 30], is used to counterbalance this effect. They were developed to reproduce the cornea with its typical shape and the endothelium with cell sizes of approximately 20 μm in diameter. These standard samples consist of a layer of polystyrene beads of calibrated diameter deposited on the internal surface of a poly(methyl-methacrylate) lens simulating the cornea. Images of the polystyrene beads must be taken in the same configurations and at the same angle of observation as in vivo pachymetry or endothelial analyses. The comparison between expected thickness and expected bead density and measured values determines the corrective factor for in vivo thickness and ECD measurements. Concerning the expected bead density corresponding to a hexagonal bead packing, the number of beads per unit area (density δ of beads) can be calculated as

$$\delta = \frac{1}{2\sqrt{3}r^2} \tag{6}$$

where r is the radius of each bead. The beads proposed in Ref. [22] have radius, r = 10.14 μm, so that the expected density δ can be calculated by Eq. (6) to be 2808 mm^{-2}.

6. In vivo results

After the calibration, corneal central thickness, ECD, HEX, and CoV were measured in vivo in a small group of ten healthy subjects (age: 20–30 years). They were enrolled on a voluntary basis following the Declaration of Helsinki. Inclusion criteria were the absence of any known corneal pathology and to be between the ages of 20 and 30 years.

The analysis was performed on the right eye of each subject, each of whom was asked to look at a far target during the image acquisitions. Images were taken with a relatively narrow slit (pachymetry) and with a larger slit to observe the endothelial mosaic (endothelial microscopy). Images were taken in the central portion of the cornea, at a distance lower than 2 mm from the center of the pupil.

Although the group is small and it might not therefore account for a reliable statistical analysis, the mean (±standard deviation) of the ten measured values was calculated. The mean central corneal thickness was found to be 502 μm (± 73 μm). The results are in reasonable agreement with data reported in the literature. For example, Olsen and Ehlers reported a mean central corneal thickness of (515 ± 33) μm calculated on 115 eyes between 10 and 90 years [32]. Doughty and Zaman [33] reported a value of 534 μm for "normal" human central corneal thickness. Wirbelauer et al. [34] found (541 ± 43) μm for the mean central corneal thickness of 108 subjects (age range: 25–87 years). Altay et al. [35] reported mean values on 137 subjects (age range: 18–64 years) equal to (522 ± 34), (543 ± 34), and (538 ± 35) μm, measured by Scheimpflug camera, specular microscopy, and ultrasound pachymetry, respectively. Compared to other techniques, the measurement of corneal thickness with the slit-lamp biomicroscope adds no extra costs for the clinicians, who routinely use this instrument. It should be noted that the method of specular reflection can only be used on subjects with healthy corneas. Keratoconus, corneal opacities, and other irregularities may distort the light beam or dim the endothelium reflex beyond acceptable levels. This disadvantage is also relevant for other techniques such as the systems based on Scheimpflug camera.

Regarding the endothelial mosaic, the mean ($\pm$ standard deviation) of ten measured values yielded 2671 mm^{-2} ($\pm$ 133 mm^{-2}) for ECD, 46% ($\pm$ 5%) for HEX, and 31% ($\pm$ 3%) for CoV. The results are in reasonable agreement with data in the literature. Variations of ECD, HEX, and CoV are expected due to several factors such as hypoxia [36] and age [20]. If considering only in vivo measurements and relatively young subjects, values of mean central ECD reported in the literature can be found in the range of 2600–3000 mm^{-2} [19, 20, 37, 38]. Central HEX measured by Wiffen et al. [19] and Zheng et al. [38] is (63 ± 7) and (49 ± 13)%. Normal CoV range is considered 20–30% [20]. As already mentioned in the introduction, endothelium analysis is often carried out by automatic instruments; however, the analysis by a digital slit-lamp biomicroscope is less expensive and allows to observe any specific region of interest of the cornea in the center and in the periphery.

7. Conclusions

A high-resolution digital sensor was applied to a Visionix VX75 slit-lamp biomicroscope. A software for image acquisition, including a live digital magnification facility, was developed. A procedure is here proposed to use the apparatus in configuration of specular reflection for pachymetry analyses and for endothelial microscopy analysis at angular magnification 36×. Images are suitable for morphometric analysis of the cell mosaic of corneal endothelium, and an automatized sequence for image analysis was developed. The effects of (i) the dioptric power of the anterior corneal surface, (ii) oblique observation, and (iii) intrinsic asymmetry of digital biomicroscopes are discussed. For a quantitative analysis of corneal thickness and endothelial cell density, these effects must be taken into consideration and can be corrected by a procedure of calibration. On the contrary, the other two parameters (endothelium cell hexagonality and coefficient of variation of the cell areas) are not influenced by these aspects.

Acknowledgements

Visionix is acknowledged for supplying a Visionix VX75 slit-lamp biomicroscope.

Conflict of interest

The authors declare no conflicts of interest.

Author details

Silvia Tavazzi[1,2*], Alessandra Parodi[1], Sara Colciago[1], Gabriele Nigrotti[2], Simone Borghesi[3] and Fabrizio Zeri[1,2,4]

1 Department of Materials Science, University of Milano Bicocca, Milan, Italy

2 COMiB Research Centre in Optics and Optometry, University of Milano Bicocca, Milan, Italy

3 Department of Mathematics and Applications, University of Milano Bicocca, Milan, Italy

4 School of Life and Health Sciences, Aston University, Birmingham, UK

*Address all correspondence to: silvia.tavazzi@unimib.it

References

[1] Agarwal T, Bhartiya S, Dada T, Panda A, Jhanji V, Yu M. Agreement of corneal thickness measurement using slit-lamp and ultrasound pachymetry. Eye & Contact Lens: Science & Clinical Practice. 2012;**38**:231-233

[2] Hitzenberger CK. Measurement of corneal thickness by low coherence interferometry. Applied Optics. 1992;**31**: 6637-6642

[3] Hitzenberger CK, Baumgartner A, Drexler W, Fercher AF. Interferometric measurement of corneal thickness with micrometer precision. American Journal of Ophthalmology. 1994;**118**:468-476

[4] Drexler W, Baumgartner A, Findl O, Hitzenberger CK, Sattmann H, Fercher AF. Submicrometer precision biometry of the anterior segment of the human eye. Investigative Ophthalmology & Visual Science. 1997;**38**:1304-1313

[5] Böhnke M, Chavanne P, Gianotti R, Salathé RP. Continuous noncontact corneal pachymetry with a high speed reflectometer. Journal of Refractive Surgery. 1998;**14**:140-146

[6] Waelti R, Böhnke M, Gianotti R, Bonvin P, Ballif JJ, Dalathé RP. Rapid and precise in vivo measurement of human corneal thickness with optical low-coherence reflectometry in normal human eyes. Journal of Biomedical Optics. 1998;**3**:253-258

[7] Huang D, Wang I, Lin CP, Puliafito CA, Fujimoto JG. Micron-resolution ranging of cornea anterior chamber by optical reflectometry. Lasers in Surgery and Medicine. 1991;**11**:419-425

[8] Izatt JA, Hee MR, Swanson EA, Lin CP, Huang D, Schuman JS, et al. Micrometer-scale resolution imaging of the anterior eye in vivo with optical coherence tomography. Archives of Ophthalmology. 1994;**112**:1584-1589

[9] Fujioka M, Nakamura M, Tatsumi Y, Kusuhara A, Maeda H, Negi A. Comparison of Pentacam Scheimpflug camera with ultrasound pachymetry and noncontact specular microscopy in measuring central corneal thickness. Current Eye Research. 2007;**32**:89-94

[10] Uçakhan OO, Ozkan M, Kanpolat A. Corneal thickness measurements in normal and keratoconic eyes: Pentacam comprehensive eye scanner versus noncontact specular microscopy and ultrasound pachymetry. Journal of Cataract and Refractive Surgery. 2006; **32**:970-977

[11] Kawana K, Tokunaga T, Miyata K, Okamoto F, Kiuchi T, Oshika T. Comparison of corneal thickness measurements using Orbscan II, non-contact specular microscopy, and ultrasonic pachymetry in eyes after laser in situ keratomileusis. The British Journal of Ophthalmology. 2004;**88**: 466-468

[12] Borrego-Sanz L, Sáenz-Francés F, Bermudez-Vallecilla M, Morales-Fernández L, Martinez-de-la Casa JM, Santos-Bueso E, et al. Agreement between central corneal thickness measured using Pentacam, ultrasound pachymetry, specular microscopy and optic biometer lenstar LS 900 and influence of ıntraocular pressure. Ophthalmologica. 2014;**231**:226-235

[13] De Bernardo M, Borelli M, Mariniello M, Lanza M, Rosa N. Pentacamvs SP3000P specular microscopy in measuring corneal thickness. Contact Lens & Anterior Eye. 2015;**38**:21-27

[14] Sanchis-Gimeno JA, Herrera M, Lleo-Perez A, Alonso L, Rahhal MS, Martinez-Soriano F. Quantitative anatomical differences in central corneal thickness values determined with scanning-slit corneal topography and

noncontact specular microscopy. Cornea. 2006;**25**:203-205

[15] Tai LY, Khaw KW, Ng CM, Subrayan V. Central corneal thickness measurements with different imaging devices and ultrasound pachymetry. Cornea. 2013;**32**:766-771

[16] Waring GO, Bourne WM, Edelhauser HF, Kenion KR. The corneal endothelium: Normal and pathologic structure and function. Ophthalmology. 1982;**89**:531-590

[17] MacRae SM, Matsuta M, Shellans S, Rich LF. The effects of hard and soft contact lenses on the corneal endothelium. American Journal of Ophthalmology. 1986;**102**:50-57

[18] Schoessler JP. Contact lens wear and the corneal endothelium. Journal of the American Optometric Association. 1987; **58**:804-810

[19] Wiffen SJ, Hodge DO, Bourne WM. The effect of contact lens wear on the central and peripheral corneal endothelium. Cornea. 2000;**19**:47-51

[20] McCarey BE, Edelhauser HF, Lynn MJ. Review of corneal endothelial specular microscopy for FDA clinical trials of refractive procedures, surgical devices and new intraocular drugs and solutions. Cornea. 2008;**27**:1-16

[21] Comanducci D, Colombo C. Vision-based magnification of corneal endothelium frames. In: Proceedings of the 9th International Conference on Computer Vision Systems ICVS'13; St. Petersburg, Russia; 2013. pp. 52-61

[22] Ferraro L, Cozza F, Scialdone A, Borghesi A, Tavazzi S. Morphometric analyses by a new slit-lamp endothelial biomicroscope. Cornea. 2016;**35**: 1347-1354

[23] Brennan NA, Smith G, Macdonald JA, Bruce AS. Theoretical principles of optical pachymetry. Ophthalmic & Physiological Optics. 1989;**9**:247-254

[24] Marelli A, De Vita IR, Cozza F, Tavazzi S. Criticality of the measurement of corneal thickness in specular reflection by digital biomicroscope. Contact Lens & Anterior Eye. 2018;**41**:531-537

[25] Patel S. Refractive index of the mammalian cornea and its influence during pachometry. Ophthalmic & Physiological Optics. 1987;**7**:503-506

[26] Schoessler J, Woloschak M. Corneal endothelium in veteran PMMA contact lenses wearers. International Contact Lens Clinic. 1981;**8**:19-25

[27] Rao GN, Lohman LE, Aquavella JV. Cell size-shape relationship in corneal endothelium. Investigative Ophthalmology & Visual Science. 1982; **22**:271-274

[28] Suda T. Mosaic pattern changes in human corneal endothelium with age. Japanese Journal of Ophthalmology. 1984;**28**:331-338

[29] Orsborn GN, Schoessler JP. Corneal endothelial polymegathism after the extended wear of rigid gas-permeable contact lenses. American Journal of Optometry and Physiological Optics. 1988;**65**:84-90

[30] Tufo S, Prazzoli E, Ferraro L, Cozza F, Borghesi A, Tavazzi S. Variable-size bead layer as standard reference for endothelial microscopes. Cornea. 2017; **36**:236-240

[31] Doughty MJ, Fonn D, Nguyen KT. Assessment of the reliability of calculations of the coefficients of variations for normal and polymegethous human corneal endothelium. Optometry and Vision Science. 1993;**70**:759-770

[32] Olsen T, Ehlers N. The thickness of the human cornea as determined by a specular method. Acta Ophthalmologica. 1984;**62**:859-871

[33] Doughty MJ, Zaman ML. Human corneal thickness and its impact on intraocular pressure measures: A review and meta-analysis approach. Survey of Ophthalmology. 2000;**44**:367-408

[34] Wirbelauer C, Scholz C, Hoerauf H, Pham DT, Laqua H, Birngruber R. Noncontact corneal pachymetry with slit lamp-adapted optical coherence tomography. American Journal of Ophthalmology. 2002;**133**:444-450

[35] Altay Y, Balta O, Demirok G, Burcu A, Balta OB, Ornek F. Agreement between corneal thickness measurements using Pentacam Scheimpflug camera, noncontact specular microscopy, and ultrasonographic pachymetry in diabetic patients. Current Eye Research. 2017;**42**:187-194

[36] Polse KA, Brand RJ, Cohen SR, Guillon M. Hypoxic effects on corneal morphology and function. Investigative Ophthalmology & Visual Science. 1990; **31**:1542-1554

[37] Amann J, Holley GP, Lee SB, et al. Increased endothelial cell density in the paracentral and peripheral regions of the human cornea. American Journal of Ophthalmology. 2003;**135**:584-590

[38] Zheng T, Le Q, Hong J, et al. Comparison of human corneal cell density by age and corneal location: An in vivo confocal microscopy study. BMC Ophthalmology. 2016;**16**:109

Section 2

Intraoperative Imaging Systems

Chapter 2

Intraoperative Optical Coherence Tomography

Samet Gulkas and Osman Cekic

Abstract

Recently, surgical instruments and imaging technology in ophthalmology have shown a great improvement. However, advances in the field of the operating microscope technology still remained unchanged with the various limitations for the surgeons. Invention of optical coherence tomography (OCT) led to a revolution in the diagnosis and monitoring of numerous anterior and posterior segment pathologies. Recently, OCT has been introduced into the operating room with an impact on the surgeons. In this chapter, we review the evolution of OCT for intraoperative use with its feasibility, surgical impacts, and limitations.

Keywords: intraoperative optical coherence tomography, microscope-integrated, anterior segment *i*OCT, posterior segment *i*OCT

1. Introduction

Optical coherence tomography (OCT) is a rapid, noninvasive, noncontact, and cross-sectional imaging method that produces images of ocular tissues. OCT uses reflected light to obtain the images from the different layers on the ocular tissues that produce different backscattered lights [1]. After using of spectral-domain OCT (SD-OCT) instead of time-domain OCT (TD-OCT), the images produced by OCT have become with higher resolution; thus, OCT has begun to provide more detailed information on ophthalmologic diagnoses [2]. Recent developments in ocular imaging technology have made the OCT a vital diagnostic tool in patient care. More recently, the availability of OCT during surgery has begun to be discussed. The introduction of OCT into the operating room (OR) called as intraoperative OCT (*i*OCT) has provided new insights into the surgical management during ophthalmic surgeries.

2. Intraoperative OCT

A number of researchers have examined the potential role of *i*OCT in various conditions and procedures, such as macular hole (MH), epiretinal membrane (ERM), retinal detachment surgery, and lamellar keratoplasty [3–6]. However, conventional clinical OCT devices are large and not portable; therefore, it would be difficult and impractical to transfer the conventional OCTs into OR. In addition, the supine position of the patient during a surgery and changes to surgical flow are other potential obstacles for image acquisition with good quality. All these hurdles forced researchers to produce a portable OCT device. Initial attempts with intraoperative OCT indicated successful results in imaging of excised tumors, postmortem specimens, structural changes after laser surgery, and in vitro human arteries and nerves [7–10]. Early investigations with *i*OCT were based on time-domain technology. Nevertheless, these investigations resulted in suboptimal image quality due to lower sensitivity and speed than novel technologies of SD-OCT and swept-source OCT (SS-OCT). In recent years, to overcome suboptimal imaging during surgeries, researchers have discovered the microscope-integrated OCT devices (MIOCTs). So far, a short overview about the evolution of *i*OCT devices was introduced. The following section will discuss various *i*OCT systems and devices and their technologies.

2.1 Intraoperative OCT systems and devices

*i*OCT devices can be classified into two main categories: portable OCT during surgical pauses and microscope-integrated OCT (MIOCT). Subsequently, portable OCTs have three subgroups: handheld, external-mounted, and microscope-mounted. On the other hand, MIOCTs have two subgroups: live two-dimensional (2D) OCT imaging and live four-dimensional (4D) OCT imaging (**Tables 1** and **2**).

2.1.1 Portable OCT devices

Portable OCT devices were the beginning step for *i*OCT. There are two basic portable systems in the literature: the Bioptigen EnVisu (Bioptigen, Research Triangle Park, NC/Leica, Wetzlar, Germany) and the Optovue iVue (Optovue, Fremont, CA, USA) [6, 11–13]. These devices can be used with the systems, including handheld, external-mounted, and microscope-mounted for image acquisition.

Handheld imaging was the first examples of the portable OCTs [11, 14]. This system has a compact handheld imaging probe connected over flexible optical fiber to a portable device. In spite of restrictions on image reproducibility and optimal aiming with the device, handheld imaging can present a good image quality. Moreover, unlike clinic tabletop OCT devices, handheld OCT has no requirement upright and cooperative patient situation. Nevertheless, the need to protect the sterile surgical field and the occurrence of motion artifacts due to instability are examples of several handicaps of handheld OCT. More importantly, the main disadvantage of handheld OCT is that it is limited to surgical pauses because of the need to remove the microscope from the patient during imaging. Unfortunately, it is impossible to obtain images of the structural changes that ensued from live tissue-instrument interactions during surgery.

System	OCT technology	Speed, resolution, wavelength	Primary visualization modes	Modes of operation	Commercial status
Optovue iVue	Spectral domain	26k, 5 lm, 840 nm	B-scans, volumes, en face on external monitor	Mounted onto stabilizing arm	FDA approved
Bioptigen Envisu	Spectral domain	17–32k†, 3–5† lm, 870 nm	B-scans, en face on external monitor	Handheld, mounted onto microscope	FDA approved

[a]*Speed is listed in terms of A-scans/second; resolution refers to axial resolution; wavelength refers to the central wavelength of the source.*
†*Not specified in publications. Range provided by manufacturer.*

Table 1.
System specifications and features of commercial HHOCT systems used in human retinal surgery to date.[a] *With the permission of Carrasco-Zevallos OM et al. under the license of CC licensing [23].*

System	OCT technology	Speed, resolution, wavelength	Primary visualization modes	OCT acquisition and features	Commercial status
Haag-Streit surgical *i*OCT	Spectral domain	10k, 10 lm, 840 nm	Live B-scans on binocular, monoscopic HUD	OCT operator control, surgeon control of OCT display via foot pedal, optical zoom	FDA approved
Zeiss Rescan 700	Spectral domain	27k, 5.5 lm, 840 nm	Live B-scans on monocular, monoscopic HUD	OCT operator control with tracking, surgeon control of OCT scan location via foot pedal	FDA approved
Bioptigen EnFocus	Spectral domain	32k, 4 lm, 860 nm	Live B-scans, static en face on external monitor	OCT operator control, surgeon control via foot pedal	FDA approved

[a]*Speed is listed in terms of A-scans/second; resolution refers to axial resolution; wavelength refers to the central wavelength of the source.*

Table 2.
System specifications and features of all commercial MIOCT systems used in human retinal surgery to date.[a] *With the permission of Carrasco-Zevallos OM et al. under the license of CC licensing [23].*

Mounting systems for the portable OCT systems were developed to address most of the handheld imaging. These external mounts contribute more stability, yet these systems require a supplementary footprint and place in the operating room [4, 6]. The microscope holders allow the surgeon to attach the portable probe directly to the microscope body, thus providing more stability than handheld imaging. Microscope foot pedal controls make it possible to control the probe position with X-Y-Z foot pedals. This foot pedal control makes easier imaging with improved image repeatability [4].

Unfortunately, the main disadvantage of portable OCTs is that it is limited to surgical pauses because of the need to remove the microscope from the patient during imaging. In other words, it is impossible to obtain images of the structural changes that ensued from live tissue-instrument interactions during surgery.

2.1.2 Microscope-integrated OCT devices

A step-by-step initiative in the *i*OCT has been the integration of OCT into microscope optics called MIOCT. Leica (Leica, Wetzlar, Germany) and Zeiss (Carl Zeiss Meditec, Oberkochen, Germany) were the first examples of these systems. In the Zeiss adaptation, a modified Cirrus (Carl Zeiss Meditec) and a modified Visante (Carl Zeiss Meditec) OCT system integrated into Zeiss microscope optical path for the posterior and anterior segment imaging, respectively, were used [3, 15, 16]. These two systems allow surgeons for real-time imaging by visualizing the instrument-tissue interaction. On the other hand, these two systems bring with it new software requirements, the need for heads-up image acquisition, and the compatibility of OCT with the surgical instrument used during imaging. Additionally, surgical maneuvers during the surgery also require Z-axis stabilization and automated tracking system to improve image quality. After the investigation of first MIOCT systems, three commercial systems were identified. Zeiss Rescan 700 was defined as the first FDA-approved MIOCT system. This system is integrated into the Zeiss Lumera 700 microscope platform. Zeiss Rescan 700 was also integrated into the microscope foot pedal system to provide surgeon targeting, orientation control. More importantly, Zeiss Rescan 700 has the first MIOCT having Z-tracking system [17, 18]. The second FDA-approved MIOCT system was the Haag-Streit MIOCT system (Haag-Streit, Koeniz, Switzerland). This system consists of a side port using OPMedT (OPMedT, Lübeck, Germany) OCT system. This system has not only a microscope-mounted viewing but also a heads-up screen too [19]. Unlike Zeiss Rescan, the Haag-Streit Surgical *i*OCT has no control system with Z-tracking; differently, this system has an optical zoom. The third commercially available and FDA-approved MIOCT system was Bioptigen EnFocus iOCT system. This system can be adapted to both Leica and Zeiss microscopes. The system has a 4-μm resolution and a different static en face on external monitor as a visualization mode. Dissimilarly, Bioptigen EnFocus system has an essential long-fiber that provides more flexibility to insert the OCT device and its computer inside the operating room (**Figure 1**) [20].

With regard to limitations of the MIOCT devices, while a volumetric data could be obtained, acquisition of the volume is slow, and volume analysis as well as visualization has necessitated comprehensive postprocessing. Another important limitation of MIOCT devices is an inefficient display of continuous instrument movement due to intraoperative real-time visualization limited by B-scans. In other words, intraocular instruments used during live surgery generally give rise to shadows on the underlying tissue in B-scan mode. This issue requires alignment of the surgical maneuvers with the B-scan to eliminate instrumental ghosting during surgery. Ehlers et al. [21] described and characterized this shadowing effect with ex vivo porcine eye surgeries. Regarding surgical instrument shading, some authors have suggested the idea of an automated instrument tracking system using a stereo camera pair [22].

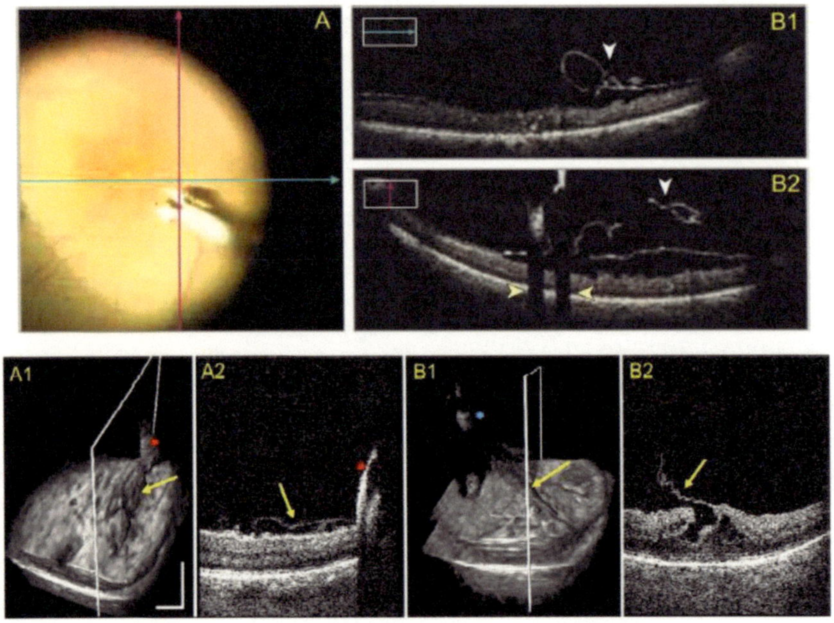

Figure 1.
Live 2D MIOCT imaging of human retinal surgery with the commercially available Rescan 700 and a Cirrus HD-OCT system adapted to an operating microscope. (A) Frame captured with the camera that records the surgeon's view through the operating microscope. The orthogonal arrows correspond to the B-scan locations. (B) Horizontal (B1) and vertical (B2) B-scans acquired with the Rescan 700 during inner limiting membrane (ILM) peeling. The membrane edge (white arrowheads) is clearly visible in the B-scans along with "shadowing" (yellow arrowheads) from the intraocular forceps. With the permission of Carrasco-Zevallos OM et al. under the license of CC licensing [23].

All real-time MIOCTs described above were limited to B-scan due to involvement of SD-OCT system having slower A-scan rate. Carrasco-Zevallos et al. [23] were the first authors who described the volumetric *i*OCT imaging of live model eye surgery. They presented a custom ultrafast SS-OCT system operating at 100 kHz of A-scan rate. This speed was three to five times faster than previous MIOCT devices. A software called a special graphics-processing unit was simultaneously used to get, process, and render volumes. Later, the same authors developed a custom microscope-integrated heads-up display (HUD) unit for stereoscopic imaging of MIOCT volumes [24, 25]. SS-MIOCT and stereoscopic HUD together were called as 4D MIOCT. In 2015, 4D MIOCT was first demonstrated by Carrasco-Zevallos et al. [23] for imaging of human retinal surgery. The volumetric frame rate varied 3.3–10 volumes per second during the surgery. Through a special mode "stream saving," OCT volumes were saved, and thus continuous volumetric recording could be acquired in the surgery. Visualization of the stereoscopic volumes by the HUD was enabled, and the surgeon could control the volume rendering via a foot pedal joystick.

Although 4D MIOCT devices have faster scan rate than 2D MIOCT due to faster A-scan rate, it requires faster A-scan rate as well as human flicker fusion rate (16 Hz) to attain optimal lateral resolution. In addition to that, instrumental shading effect is still one of the major limitations in 4D MIOCT as well in 2D MIOCT devices.

2.2 Clinical applications of intraoperative OCT

In this part of the chapter, we will provide information on the clinical use of *i*OCT. In terms of both anterior and posterior segments, there are numerous of clinical studies related to feasibility and real-time assessment of the surgical feedback during the anterior and posterior surgeries [4–6, 11, 13, 14, 16–18, 20]. The two most important prospective clinical studies are the PIONNER study and the DISCOVER study [4, 20]. In these studies, the portable microscope-mounted *i*OCT in the PIONNER study (n = 531) and the microscope-integrated *i*OCT in the DISCOVER study (n = 227) were evaluated. There are not only large-scale prospective but also numerous smaller clinical studies in the literature. In the section that follows, feasibility and efficacy of *i*OCT for the anterior segment applications will be argued.

2.2.1 Anterior segment

Intraoperative OCT has been used for various anterior segment surgeries involving penetrating and lamellar keratoplasty, cataract surgeries, and excisional biopsy procedures [4, 15, 16, 19, 22].

*i*OCT has been used for full-thickness and lamellar keratoplasty surgeries for decision-making. Particularly, *i*OCT can be very useful to evaluate in cases with extensive synechiae or iridocorneal scars. It may help to protect iris tissue from traumas during initial trephination [26]. Furthermore, the graft-host position can be estimated during surgery; thereby, it can help to construct proper graft-host relationship. In anterior lamellar keratoplasty, the presence of residual corneal opacities following microkeratome-assisted removal of anterior stromal layers can be detected, and their extensions may be easily confirmed by *i*OCT. Again, the thickness of residual stromal bed can be assessed, thus increasing the safety of operation [27]. As is known, it is very important to maintain an intact descemet membrane (DM) during deep anterior lamellar keratoplasty (DALK), and large bubble technique is widely used for this purpose. The *i*OCT helps to confirm the presence of large bubbles, detect subclinical large bubbles, and conduct additional dissections. In addition to these, the presence of any interface fluid can be determined with the help of the *i*OCT, thus helping to determine the extra maneuvers that need to be done to ensure proper position of tissues to the end of the surgery. However, the instrumental shadowing effect may hinder the visualization of the underlying structures, thereby limiting the effective use of *i*OCT during intrastromal insertion of the needle. Therefore, surgical pause is necessary to evaluate the underlying tissues [17, 28, 29]. *i*OCT is a helpful intraoperative imaging method not only in full-thickness and lamellar but also in endothelial keratoplasty applications, e.g., descemet stripping automated endothelial keratoplasty (DSAEK) and descemet membrane endothelial keratoplasty (DMEK). Especially, in double-pass technique in DSAEK, the residual donor thickness following the first microkeratome passing can be easily determined with guiding *i*OCT to select of ideal blade size for the next microkeratome passing. This will minimize the chance of perforation of donor tissue by obtaining very thin donor lenticules [30]. Additionally, *i*OCT provides an advantage to identify and remove the descemet membrane in case of extreme edematous corneas. Furthermore, *i*OCT allows a continuous monitoring during the graft insertion and unfolding process. In DMEK, *i*OCT is a very convenient tool to provide faster graft orientation and position, especially in cases with edematous cornea [31]. In the DISCOVER study, it was reported that the surgeons required additional surgical maneuvers in 41% of the cases having DSAEK [18]. Similarly, in the PIONNER study, results showed that 19% of the cases in which surgeons believed the graft was completely apposed had still persistent fluid detected in the *i*OCT; hence, it would require more maneuvers and vice versa; in 47% of cases where the surgeon believed the graft to be partially apposed, there was complete apposition in *i*OCT imaging [4]. These two studies have also revealed that *i*OCT aids changes in dissection depth in 38–56% of cases [4, 20]. Briefly, it can be concluded that *i*OCT in keratoplasty procedures can minimize unnecessary manipulations and surgical time.

Recently, *i*OCT has been used in various stages of a cataract surgery. The wound structure, status of posterior capsule, and position of intraocular lens (IOL) can be easily assessed via *i*OCT during a cataract surgery [32]. In a case report, it was reported that MIOCT was a very feasible tool to evaluate the wound architecture, integrity of the posterior capsule, IOL position, and efficacy of stromal hydration. The authors suggested that *i*OCT could be helpful in real-time early detection of various complications of cataract surgery, thus allowing the surgeon to manage the complication immediately [33].

More recently, in taking biopsy and excisional procedures, such as retrocorneal fibrosis and pterygium excision, and evaluating intraoperative changes in corneal structure during excimer laser phototherapeutic keratectomy, feasibility of *i*OCT was assessed, and the results were promising [34, 35].

2.2.2 Posterior segment

Similar to the use of *i*OCT for anterior segment surgery, *i*OCT has a wide range of potentials for posterior segment surgery. Numerous vitreoretinal pathologies were described with *i*OCT, such as retinopathy of premature (ROP), proliferative diabetic retinopathy, macular hole, epiretinal membrane (ERM), retinal detachment, and myopic foveoschisis [4, 5, 20, 36–39]. The *i*OCT has provided new insights into the underlying pathophysiology for some of these conditions. PIONEER and DISCOVER studies provided valuable information about *i*OCT for posterior segment surgeons [4, 20]. We will discuss the results of these studies at the end of this section.

Chavala et al. [11] reported that they identified preretinal structures and retinoschisis with *i*OCT in case of ROP. They suggested that these new findings might markedly affect the surgeons to make a decision resulting in various alterations during the operation. It is thought that *i*OCT may allow the surgeons to assess the extents of both horizontal and anteroposterior tractional structures in ROP cases; thus, the surgeons could carefully dissect or peel while sparing the other retinal structures. Additionally, *i*OCT is very useful detecting the flat neovascular fronds in ROP cases as well as other vascular retinopathies; thereby, this could prevent iatrogenic hemorrhages by determining the extent and location of the neovascular fronds during the surgery.

The *i*OCT helps the surgeon to determine the firmness of vitreomacular tractions; therefore, in case of foveal cyst, de-roofing risk would diminish, and inadvertent macular hole could be eliminated. Similarly, during an ERM and internal limiting membrane (ILM) peeling, the *i*OCT decreases the risk of inadvertent grasping of the retina while completing ERM/ILM peeling (**Figure 2**).
In a recent study, it was reported that a membrane peeling with the guidance of *i*OCT was enabled without the use of adjuvant dyes to identify of membrane edges [36]. Especially in a macular hole surgery, this advantage of *i*OCT allows visualization of the alterations in the macular hole architecture as well as in the outer retina [37, 40]. In addition, during a macular hole surgery, the surgeon may worry about inadvertent touching or tearing on nerve fiber layer. In such situation, the *i*OCT with real-time feedback can prevent inadvertent damage on nerve fiber layer.

One of the retinopathies in which the *i*OCT is used is myopic foveoschisis. As known, there are multiple layers of schisis in this retinopathy, and this involves vital dye staining to make certain that the whole cortical vitreous has been removed. However, the cases with myopic foveoschisis have a longer axial length, thus giving rise to poor dying. The *i*OCT can allow not only to better evaluate the ILM but also to prevent iatrogenic breaks by improving visualization in a myopic retina.

*i*OCT enables to provide more information in retinal detachment cases. In recent various studies, the *i*OCT revealed the presence of subclinical persistent subretinal fluid under perfluorocarbon tamponade in most of the cases undergoing retinal

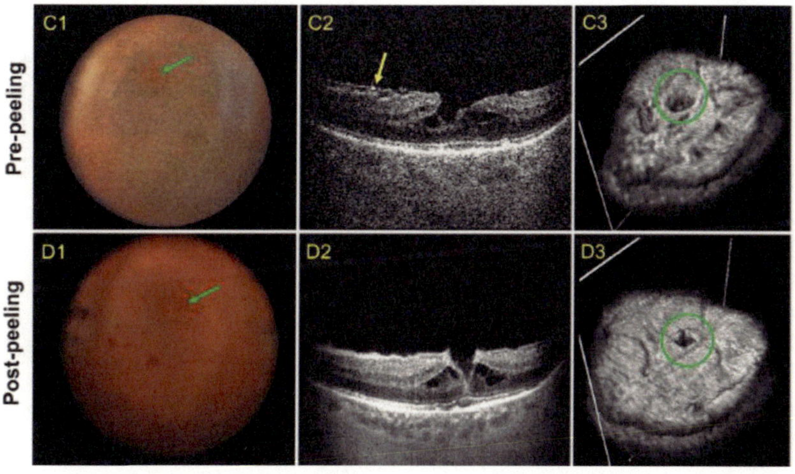

Figure 2.
*B-scan (C1) and volume (C2) acquired intraoperatively before epiretinal membrane (ERM) peeling with the reconfigured Cirrus HD-OCT system. B-scan (D1) and volume (D2) acquired after ERM peeling. The volumes required intensive postprocessing to render and were visualized postoperatively. The prepeeling volumes depict ERM and puckering of the retina, while the post-peeling volumes show a small residual part of ERM (**Figure 1**). With the permission of Carrasco-Zevallos OM et al. under the license of CC licensing [23].*

detachment operation [4, 5, 20]. Furthermore, *i*OCT can help to detect proliferative vitreoretinopathy changes and border architecture of retinal tears.

In proliferative diabetic retinopathy, *i*OCT provides an enhanced imaging during delamination of membranes. For this reason, the *i*OCT facilitates the identification of the surgical plane, which permits membrane peeling in a safe manner. In addition to that, in the cases of dense vitreous hemorrhage, *i*OCT can help to assess intra-operatively the underlying macular pathology, such as intraretinal fluid, macular edema, or presence of a membrane, which may impact the surgeon in changing operation plan [38, 39].

Recently, in the 3-year outcome reports of the DISCOVER study, the use of *i*OCT for image-guided retinal biopsy and placement of Argus II implant was reported. It was demonstrated that *i*OCT facilitates insertion of the biopsy site and enabled confirming placement of the implant in optimal location [41, 42]. More recently, a few studies reported the use of *i*OCT verifying subretinal location of gene therapy and stem cells during the operation [43, 44].

Finally, the outcomes in posterior segment surgery in the PIONNER and DISCOVER studies showed that *i*OCT identified residual membranes in 13–22% of the cases whom the surgeon believed that membrane peeling was completed; conversely, in 15–40% of the cases, the surgeon still thought the presence of residual membrane, yet *i*OCT indicated that complete removal of the membrane had been performed [4, 20]. Additionally, *i*OCT provided addition of useful data concerning surgical anatomic features in 59.4% of the cases, and the information obtaining with *i*OCT impacted the surgery in 29.2% of the cases [20].

3. Conclusion

As known, in a very short time, conventional tabletop OCT has acquired its place in practice; subsequently, real-time intraoperative feedback with the *i*OCT appears to be a revolution in the OCT technology. Up to now, overall study reports related to *i*OCT, especially the PIONNER and DISCOVER study, have enhanced our understanding of *i*OCT technology and its unique advantages in surgical efficiency. *i*OCT may lead to refine and replace conventional surgical procedures with novel procedures, so that, with this technology, improved individual surgical management and patient care can be achieved. However, this technology has still a few limitations. The overall outcomes related to feasibility of *i*OCT need to be validated with additional prospective randomized trials.

Conflict of interest

There are no conflicts of interest.

Author details

Samet Gulkas[1]* and Osman Cekic[2]

1 Sanliurfa Training and Research Hospital, Sanliurfa, Turkey

2 University of Marmara, School of Medicine, Istanbul, Turkey

*Address all correspondence to: drsametgulkas@gmail.com

References

[1] Huang D, Swanson EA, Lin CP, et al. Optical coherence tomography. Science. 1991;**254**:1178-1181

[2] Choma M, Sarunic M, Yang C, et al. Sensitivity advantage of swept source and Fourier domain optical coherence tomography. Optics Express. 2003;**11**:2183-2189

[3] Binder S, Falkner-Radler CI, Hauger C, et al. Feasibility of intrasurgical spectral-domain optical coherence tomography. Retina. 2011;**31**:1332-1336

[4] Ehlers JP, Dupps WJ, Kaiser PK, et al. The prospective intraoperative and perioperative ophthalmic ImagiNg with optical coherence tomography (PIONEER) study: 2-year results. American Journal of Ophthalmology. 2014;**158**:999-1007

[5] Ehlers JP, Ohr MP, Kaiser PK, et al. Novel microarchitectural dynamics in rhegmatogenous retinal detachments identified with intraoperative optical coherence tomography. Retina. 2013;**33**:1428-1434

[6] Ray R, Baranano DE, Fortun JA, et al. Intraoperative microscope-mounted spectral domain optical coherence tomography for evaluation of retinal anatomy during macular surgery. Ophthalmology. 2011;**118**:2212-2217

[7] Boppart SA, Bouma BE, Pitris C, et al. Intraoperative assessment of microsurgery with three-dimensional optical coherence tomography. Radiology. 1998;**208**:81-86

[8] Boppart SA, Herrmann JM, Pitris C, et al. Real-time optical coherence tomography for minimally invasive imaging of prostate ablation. Computer Aided Surgery. 2001;**6**:94-103

[9] Brezinski ME, Tearney GJ, Bouma B, et al. Optical biopsy with optical coherence tomography. Annals of the New York Academy of Sciences. 1998;**838**:68-74

[10] Shakhov AV, Terentjeva AB, Kamensky VA, et al. Optical coherence tomography monitoring for laser surgery of laryngeal carcinoma. Journal of Surgical Oncology. 2001;**77**:253-258

[11] Chavala SH, Farsiu S, Maldonado R, et al. Insights into advanced retinopathy of prematurity using handheld spectral domain optical coherence tomography imaging. Ophthalmology. 2009;**116**:2448-2456

[12] Dayani PN, Maldonado R, Farsiu S, et al. Intraoperative use of handheld spectral domain optical coherence tomography imaging in macular surgery. Retina. 2009;**29**:1457-1468

[13] Pichi F, Alkabes M, Nucci P, et al. Intraoperative SD-OCT in macular surgery. Ophthalmic Surgery, Lasers & Imaging. 2012;**43**:S54-S60

[14] Scott AW, Farsiu S, Enyedi LB, et al. Imaging the infant retina with a hand-held spectral-domain optical coherence tomography device. American Journal of Ophthalmology. 2009;**147**:364-373

[15] Hirnschall N, Amir-Asgari S, Maedel S, et al. Predicting the postoperative intraocular lens position using continuous intraoperative optical coherence tomography measurements. Investigative Ophthalmology & Visual Science. 2013;**54**:5196-5203

[16] Hirnschall N, Norrby S, Weber M, et al. Using continuous intraoperative optical coherence tomography measurements of the aphakic eye for intraocular lens power calculation. The British Journal of Ophthalmology. 2015;**99**:7-10

[17] Ehlers JP, Goshe J, Dupps WJ, et al. Determination of feasibility

and utility of microscope-integrated optical coherence tomography during ophthalmic surgery: The DISCOVER study RESCAN results. JAMA Ophthalmology. 2015;**133**:1124-1132

[18] Ehlers JP, Kaiser PK, Srivastava SK. Intraoperative optical coherence tomography using the RESCAN 700: Preliminary results from the DISCOVER study. The British Journal of Ophthalmology. 2014;**98**:1329-1332

[19] Steven P, Le Blanc C, Velten K, et al. Optimizing descemet membrane endothelial keratoplasty using intraoperative optical coherence tomography. JAMA Ophthalmology. 2013;**131**:1135-1142

[20] Ehlers JP, Modi YS, Pecen PE, et al. The DISCOVER study 3-year results: Feasibility and usefulness of microscope-integrated intraoperative OCT during ophthalmic surgery. Ophthalmology. 2018;**125**:1014-1027

[21] Ehlers JP, Tao YK, Farsiu S, et al. Integration of a spectral domain optical coherence tomography system into a surgical microscope for intraoperative imaging. Investigative Ophthalmology & Visual Science. 2011;**52**:3153-3159

[22] El-Haddad MT, Tao YK. Automated stereo vision instrument tracking for intraoperative OCT guided anterior segment ophthalmic surgical maneuvers. Biomedical Optics Express. 2015;**6**:3014-3031

[23] Carrasco-Zevallos OM, Keller B, Viehland C, et al. Optical coherence tomography for retinal surgery: Perioperative analysis to real-time four-dimensional image-guided surgery. Investigative Ophthalmology & Visual Science. 2016;**57**:OCT37-OCT50

[24] Shen L, Carrasco-Zevallos O, Keller B, et al. Novel microscope-integrated stereoscopic heads-up display for intrasurgical optical coherence tomography. Biomedical Optics Express. 2016;**7**:1711-1726

[25] Tao YK, Ehlers JP, Toth CA, et al. Intraoperative spectral domain optical coherence tomography for vitreoretinal surgery. Optics Letters. 2010;**35**:3315-3317

[26] Eguchi H, Kusaka S, Arimura-Koike E, et al. Intraoperative optical coherence tomography (RESCAN((R)) 700) for detecting iris incarceration and iridocorneal adhesion during keratoplasty. International Ophthalmology. 2017;**37**:761-765

[27] Titiyal JS, Kaur M, Falera R. Intraoperative optical coherence tomography in anterior segment surgeries. Indian Journal of Ophthalmology. 2017;**65**:116-121

[28] Au J, Goshe J, Dupps WJ Jr, et al. Intraoperative optical coherence tomography for enhanced depth visualization in deep anterior lamellar keratoplasty from the PIONEER study. Cornea. 2015;**34**:1039-1043

[29] Steven P, Le Blanc C, Lankenau E, et al. Optimising deep anterior lamellar keratoplasty (DALK) using intraoperative online optical coherence tomography (iOCT). The British Journal of Ophthalmology. 2014;**98**:900-904

[30] Kobayashi A, Yokogawa H, Mori N, et al. Visualization of precut DSAEK and pre-stripped DMEK donor corneas by intraoperative optical coherence tomography using the RESCAN 700. BMC Ophthalmology. 2016;**16**:135

[31] Saad A, Guilbert E, Grise-Dulac A, et al. Intraoperative OCT-assisted DMEK: 14 consecutive cases. Cornea. 2015;**34**:802-807

[32] Das S, Kummelil MK, Kharbanda V, et al. Microscope integrated intraoperative spectral domain optical coherence tomography for cataract

surgery: Uses and applications. Current Eye Research. 2016;**41**:643-652

[33] Almutlak MA, Aloniazan T, May W. Real-time optical coherence tomography incorporated in the operating microscope during cataract surgery. Middle East African Journal of Ophthalmology. 2017;**24**:156-158

[34] Ruland K, Bouldin TW, Davis RM, et al. Intraoperative optical coherence tomography-assisted retrocorneal fibrous membrane biopsy and excision. American Journal of Ophthalmology Case Reports. 2018;**11**:101-104

[35] Siebelmann S, Horstmann J, Scholz P, et al. Intraoperative changes in corneal structure during excimer laser phototherapeutic keratectomy (PTK) assessed by intraoperative optical coherence tomography. Graefe's Archive for Clinical and Experimental Ophthalmology. 2018;**256**:575-581

[36] Falkner-Radler CI, Glittenberg C, Gabriel M, et al. Intrasurgical microscope-integrated spectral domain optical coherence tomography-assisted membrane peeling. Retina. 2015;**35**:2100-2106

[37] Xu D, Yuan A, Kaiser PK, et al. A novel segmentation algorithm for volumetric analysis of macular hole boundaries identified with optical coherence tomography. Investigative Ophthalmology & Visual Science. 2013;**54**:163-169

[38] Ehlers JP, Griffith JF, Srivastava SK. Intraoperative optical coherence tomography during vitreoretinal surgery for dense vitreous hemorrhage in the pioneer study. Retina. 2015;**35**:2537-2542

[39] Khan M, Srivastava SK, Reese JL, et al. Intraoperative OCT-assisted surgery for proliferative diabetic retinopathy in the DISCOVER study. Ophthalmology Retina. 2018;**2**:411-417

[40] Itoh Y, Vasanji A, Ehlers JP. Volumetric ellipsoid zone mapping for enhanced visualisation of outer retinal integrity with optical coherence tomography. The British Journal of Ophthalmology. 2016;**100**:295-299

[41] Browne AW, Ehlers JP, Sharma S, et al. Intraoperative optical coherence tomography-assisted chorioretinal biopsy in the DISCOVER study. Retina. 2017;**37**:2183-2187

[42] Rachitskaya AV, Yuan A, Marino MJ, et al. Intraoperative OCT imaging of the argus II retinal prosthesis system. Ophthalmic Surgery, Lasers and Imaging Retina. 2016;**47**:999-1003

[43] Gregori NZ, Lam BL, Davis JL. Intraoperative use of microscope-integrated optical coherence tomography for subretinal gene therapy delivery. Retina. 2017. [Epub ahead of print]

[44] Mandai M, Kurimoto Y, Takahashi M. Autologous induced stem-cell-derived retinal cells for macular degeneration. The New England Journal of Medicine. 2017;**377**:792-793

Chapter 3

Microscope-Integrated Intraoperative Optical Coherence Tomography in Retinal Surgery

Jesus Hernan Gonzalez-Cortes, Abraham Olvera-Barrios, Jesus Emiliano Gonzalez-Cantu and Jesus Mohamed-Hamsho

Abstract

Imaging techniques of the posterior segment of the eye have gradually evolved and tremendously improved during the last decade. A widespread implementation of optical coherence tomography (OCT) for the management and diagnosis of retinal conditions, with a concurrent advance in integrative technology, led to the integration of the OCT into the microscope for its intraoperative use. Regarding posterior segment eye surgery, some of the most common diagnoses in which microscope-integrated OCT (MIOCT) can result of great value are epiretinal membrane, macular hole (MH), proliferative diabetic retinopathy (PDR) and, less frequently, for inflammatory diseases, chorioretinal biopsies, and retinal implants. The impact on the surgical procedure and, possibly, on the postoperative outcome could relate to the definition of whether or not a membrane has been entirely peeled, the presence of residual membranes, and the option to perform a dissection without the need of vital dyes. The possibility of correct topographical location of hemorrhages, suspect lesions, or implants can also facilitate the surgical decision-making during biopsies or prosthesis implantation. Microscope-integrated OCT is a feasible and useful tool that can provide valuable information during surgery impact on decision-making, anatomic results, surgical safety and provide opportunity to individualize surgical treatment for each patient.

Keywords: intraoperative optical coherence tomography, retinal surgery, vitreomacular interface, membrane peeling, retinal detachment

1. Introduction

The development of microsurgery enhanced the precision with which ophthalmic surgical procedures are currently performed. Its origins date back to 1876, when the first binocular magnifying device was invented by T. Saemisch of Bonn [1]. It was not until 1953, with the manufacture of a microscope with coaxial illumination, that the use of the surgical microscope became more widely available and adapted to ocular surgery [2–4]. Three years later, in 1956, the term “microsurgery” was used for the first time by H. M. Dekking of Göningen [5]. Almost two decades before the use of binocular magnifying devices, Hermann von Helmholtz invented ophthalmoscopy in 1851 and allowed us to see, for the first time, the human retina [6]. Under this rapidly evolving background, the development of pars plana vitrectomy (PPV) in 1970 revolutionized retinal surgery with less invasive procedures and better results in terms of visual acuity and patient satisfaction [7].

In addition to the operating microscope, imaging techniques of the posterior segment of the eye have tremendously improved during the last two decades. Optical coherence tomography (OCT) became readily and more widely available during the last 10 years and has become one of the most commonly ordered diagnostic tests in ophthalmology [8–12]. The detail on the retinal architecture provided by OCT allows to better characterize, diagnose, manage, and give prognosis of a wide range of vitreoretinal conditions.

1.1 Integration of OCT into the operating theater

Further improvements in software and imaging started a new transition of this powerful technology to the operating room. Firstly, it was used as a perioperative tool to image pediatric patients, with clear limitations for image acquisition, portability, and sterility [13, 14], and then as a handheld OCT scan head: Bioptigen SDOIS/ Envisu portable system (Bioptigen, Research Triangle Park, NC) and Optovue IVue (Optovue, Fremont, CA) [15–18]. Advantages of the handheld OCT imaging are flexibility of scan head orientation and dynamic positioning of the scan during acquisition. On the other hand, disadvantages were its poor reproducibility, optimal targeting, and the surgeon learning curve [16, 17, 19–21]. A further step forward was taken with the integration of an OCT scan head to the operating microscope, a model that allowed portability, stability, repeatability, efficiency, control from the foot pedal, and an easier learning curve for surgeons [16, 17, 22–24]. However, a major drawback of this system was the need to stop the surgical procedure to image the retina: a lack of real-time imaging. The 2-year results of the Prospective Intraoperative and Perioperative Ophthalmic ImagiNg With Optical CoherEncE TomogRaphy (PIONEER) study published in 2014 [17] demonstrated the potential of this imaging tool in the operating theater. A total of 531 eyes were enrolled, from which 256 underwent posterior segment surgery. The three most frequent retinal procedures in this study were epiretinal membrane (ERM) peeling (35%), macular hole (MH) surgery (23%), and rhegmatogenous retinal detachment (RRD) repair (17%). Intraoperative OCT impacted on the surgeons' understanding of the anatomical configuration of the region of interest and/or on the surgical procedure in 43% of the cases of retinal membrane peeling and impacted on surgical decision-making in at least 13% of the procedures in which the surgeon wanted to evaluate the outcome after initial membrane peeling [17].

Microscope-integrated OCT (MIOCT) provided real-time imaging when integrative technological progress allowed to incorporate a scanner head/system which is, ideally, coaxial and parafocal with the optical system to the operating microscope [25–28]. Haag-Streit (Haag-Streit, Koeniz, Switzerland), Leica (Leica Microsystems, Buffalo Grove, IL, USA), and Zeiss (Carl Zeiss Meditec, Jena, Germany) have currently available commercial MIOCT systems: iOCT, EnFocus, and Rescan 700, respectively [29–34]. Despite outcomes are still debatable, literature reports have suggested the feasibility and potentially significant usefulness of an intraoperative MIOCT [35–38]. The 3-year results of the Determination of Feasibility of Intraoperative Spectral-Domain Microscope Combined/Integrated OCT Visualization during En Face Retinal And Ophthalmic Surgery (DISCOVER) study were published in 2018 [33]. In this report, 877 eyes were enrolled, and 593 of those underwent retinal surgery. The use of MIOCT altered surgical decision-making in 29.2% of the procedures [33].

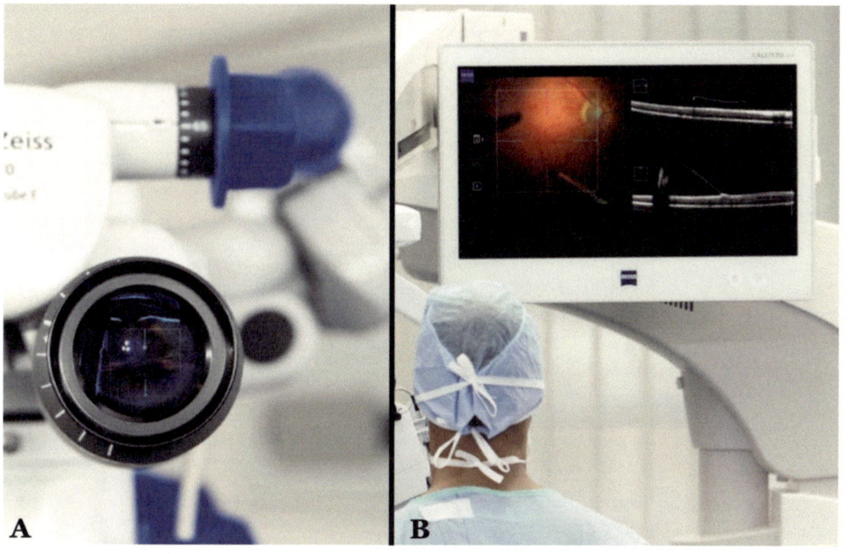

Figure 1.
Display modalities of the microscope-integrated optical coherence tomography in the ZEISS RESCAN 700. (A) Heads-up display, showing a vertical and horizontal OCT scan within the oculars. (B) An external display screen allows the surgeon to review the scans in a more detailed manner. Images courtesy of Carl Zeiss Meditec.

In order to enhance the intraoperative use of MIOCT, optimized features like automation, effective display systems, and better software analysis are required for the near future. The recent devices allow real-time and static capture acquisition of anterior and posterior segment images during surgery [31–34]. Nevertheless, they lack automation, and surgeon or assistant input can be necessary. The imaging scan is delivered to the surgeon in a dual manner: as an external display screen or a heads-up display within the oculars, providing versatility and facilitating its intraoperative use (**Figure 1**) [33]. Microscope-integrated OCT provides the surgeon with an additional tool to better evaluate the case in a real-time fashion, enhance surgical precision, and facilitate surgical decision-making.

2. Surgical implications

The intraoperative advantages of the MIOCT during surgery are wide. **Table 1** summarizes the potential surgical implications according to different pathologies.

2.1 Vitreoretinal interface disorders

Conditions comprising vitreoretinal interface disorders (MH, vitreomacular traction (VMT), and ERM) result in one of the best scenarios for the use of MIOCT [34, 35, 37, 39, 40]. Intraoperative visualization of vitreomacular interface components and alterations can potentially contribute to surgical decision-making in membrane peeling procedures, because of the readiness to obtain real-time imaging of subclinical alterations (e.g., residual membranes, retinal elevations, microarchitectural perturbations in the distances between ellipsoid zone and retinal pigment epithelium (RPE), as well as alterations of the inner retinal surface) [15–17, 33, 39–42]. The ability to perform a membrane peeling with the MIOCT could result in a reduction of the use of vital dyes, a minimization of the risk of retinal pharmacotoxicity, and a reduction of surgical time [35, 43–45].

Preoperative diagnosis	Procedure	Utility
Vitreomacular interface disorders		
Macular hole	Vitrectomy + ILM peeling	Differentiation between ERM and ILM Visualization of the ILM border Evidence or residual ILM or ERM Volumetric assessment of the retinal edges surrounding the MH Assessment of anatomical closure Potential reduction of the use of vital dyes
Vitreomacular traction syndrome		Differentiation between ERM and ILM Visualization of the ILM border Evidence or residual ILM or ERM Assessment of induced full-thickness macular or retinal holes
Epiretinal membrane		Potential reduction of the use of vital dyes
Retinal detachment	Vitrectomy	Assessment of subretinal fluid Identification of subclinical MH Delimitation of PVR and assistance during dissection Evidence of subretinal migration of heavy liquids or silicone oil Assistance in removal of subretinal heavy liquids or silicone oil
Proliferative Diabetic Retinopathy	Vitrectomy	Evidence of membranes Identification of surgical planes Delineate areas of tractive retinal detachment Topographical localization of hemorrhages (Subhyaloid, sub-ILM, subretinal) Diagnose and assess (volume and ultrastructure) of center involved or clinically significant macular edema. Assist during ILM peeling with the previously listed advantages in the section of vitreomacular interface disorders of this table.
Pediatric retinal surgery		
Retinopathy of prematurity	Examination under general anesthesia + Vitrectomy	Delineation of surgical planes Assessment of preexisting/induced full-thickness macular or retinal holes
Retinoblastoma	Examination under general anesthesia	Two-dimensional assessment of masses Identification of subretinal fluid Assessment of calcification
Shaken baby syndrome	Examination under general anesthesia +/- Vitrectomy	Assessment of full-thickness macular or retinal holes Topographical localization of hemorrhages (Subhyaloid, sub-ILM, subretinal)
Other vitreoretinal conditions		
Chorioretinal biopsy	Vitrectomy	Identification of surgical planes Delineation of normal and pathological tissue Real-time visualization of aspiration needle/surgical instruments
Retinal prostheses		Assistance during the positioning of the implant

ILM: Internal limiting membrane; ERM: Epiretinal membrane; MH: Macular hole; PVR: Proliferative vitreoretinopathy

Table 1.
Surgical implications of microscope-integrated optical coherence tomography.

2.1.1 Macular hole

The dynamic nature of the internal limiting membrane (ILM) peeling has been evidenced with MIOCT [39, 46]. Modifications of the retinal ultrastructure and geometry of MH during the ILM peeling have been described [17, 31, 42, 47–49]. Assessment of the border of the ILM peeling (**Figure 2**), residual ILM, retinal trauma (**Figure 3**), and anatomical closure (**Figure 4**) can be easily made in a real-time fashion [39, 46]. A volume increase and base area increase of MH, with a concurrent decrease in the apex height, have been evidenced following ILM peeling

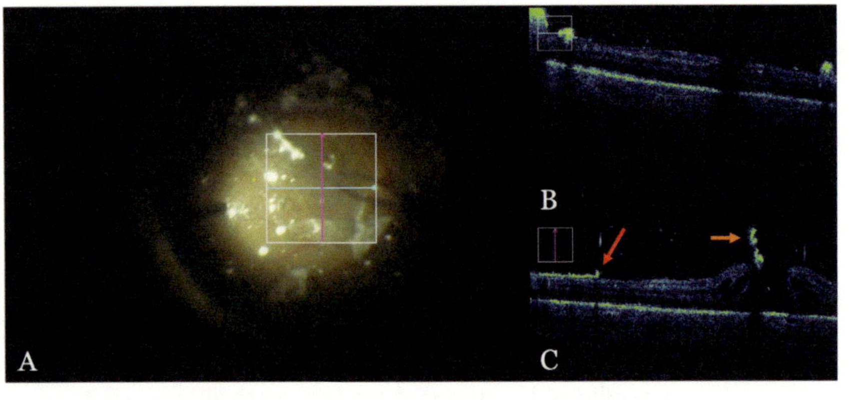

Figure 2.
Intraoperative assessment after internal limiting membrane (ILM) peeling with preservative-free triamcinolone of a macular hole (MH). (A) Color screenshot of the surgical video that delineates the area of the ILM peeling. White triamcinolone particles can be easily seen. (B) Horizontal scan just inferior to the MH. (C) the two-dimensional vertical image scan evidences the transitional zone of the ILM peeling; the red arrow demonstrates the border of the ILM tear inferiorly. Hyperreflective foci correlating with triamcinolone particles can be appreciated in the vitreous cavity, and an ILM remnant stained with triamcinolone is evidenced in the inferior border of the MH (orange arrow).

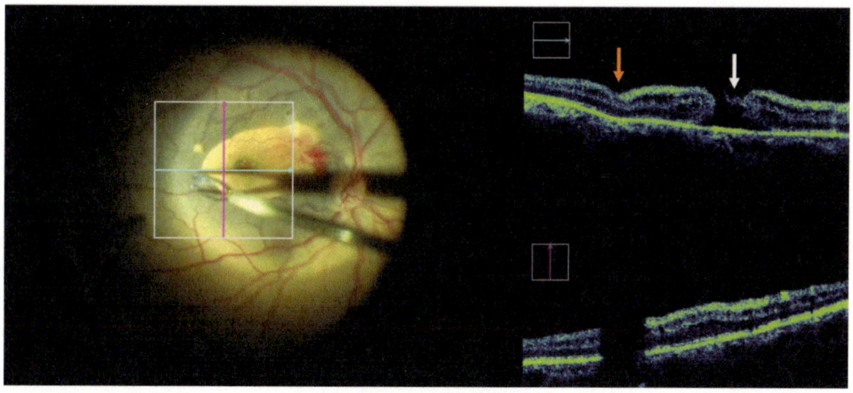

Figure 3.
Intraoperative scan after internal limiting membrane (ILM) peeling of a macular hole (MH). The imaging scan demonstrates a residual fragment of ILM in the nasal border of the MH (white arrow). Additionally, an indentation in the internal retinal layers is evidenced secondary to excessive manipulation of that area during the ILM peeling procedure (orange arrow). Preretinal hemorrhages are seen superotemporal to the optic nerve head.

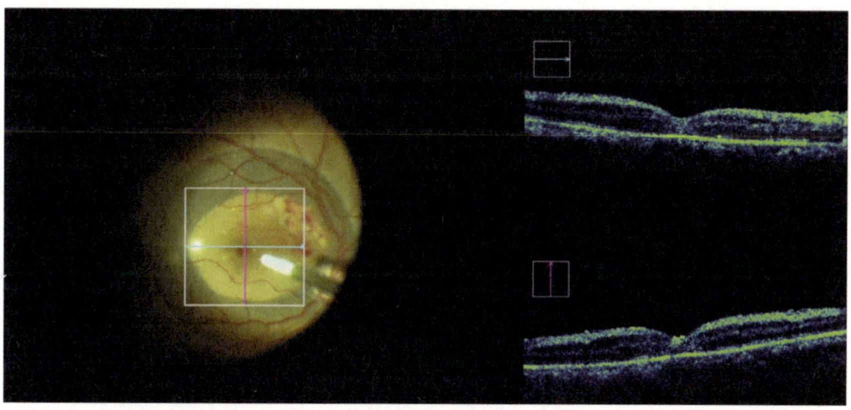

Figure 4.
Optical coherence tomography scan under the heavy liquid after internal limiting membrane (ILM) peeling. Anatomic closure was achieved after performing a gently passive suction maneuver with a 25G silicone-tipped cannula.

[39, 46, 47, 50]. Additionally, the distance between ellipsoid zone and RPE and the lateral extension of this expansion have been documented and associated with anatomical and functional outcomes [16, 17, 41, 42, 47, 50–52].

2.1.2 Vitreomacular traction syndrome

The use of MIOCT for these cases poses a potentially useful role. Release of the traction can be confirmed; dynamic anatomical modifications, changes in outer retinal relations of ellipsoid zone and EPR and residual membranes, and formations of full-thickness macular or retinal holes can be identified as well [15, 17, 20, 33].

2.1.3 Epiretinal membrane

Outer retinal modifications have also been documented following ERM and/or ILM peel in ERM. A decrease in subretinal reflectivity appreciated after these procedures correlates with a considerable expansion of the distance between the ellipsoid zone and the RPE [16, 17, 42, 47, 51]. These changes have been also associated with visual and anatomical recovery rates; however, further studies are needed to confirm this correlation [51].

2.2 Retinal detachment

The surgical benefit of real-time OCT imaging in retinal detachment (RD) repair may not be straightforward. However, intraoperative anatomical features could be relevant for the prognosis of these cases [17, 24, 33]. Additionally, complex cases with severe vitreoproliferative retinopathy could be assisted with real-time imaging and successfully addressed (**Figure 5B**). It has been evidenced that nearly all eyes undergoing surgery with perfluorocarbon liquid tamponade have some degree of subretinal fluid (**Figure 5A,B**) [24, 53]. According to the literature, foveal microarchitecture, the amount of submacular fluid, and the integrity of the ellipsoid zone following application of perfluorocarbon liquid may be of significance for the visual outcomes [17, 24, 33]. In cases where subretinal migration of perfluorocarbon liquid is present, correct visualization of the liquid bubbles and complete removal can be verified [53]. Detection of subclinical MH, occult membranes, or retinal breaks is possible with this technology, an advantage that modifies the surgical procedure and has an impact on the patient outcome [33].

2.3 Proliferative diabetic retinopathy

Vitreoretinal proliferation in diabetic retinopathy poses some of the most complex cases of vitreoretinal surgeries. The use of MIOCT can facilitate the correct

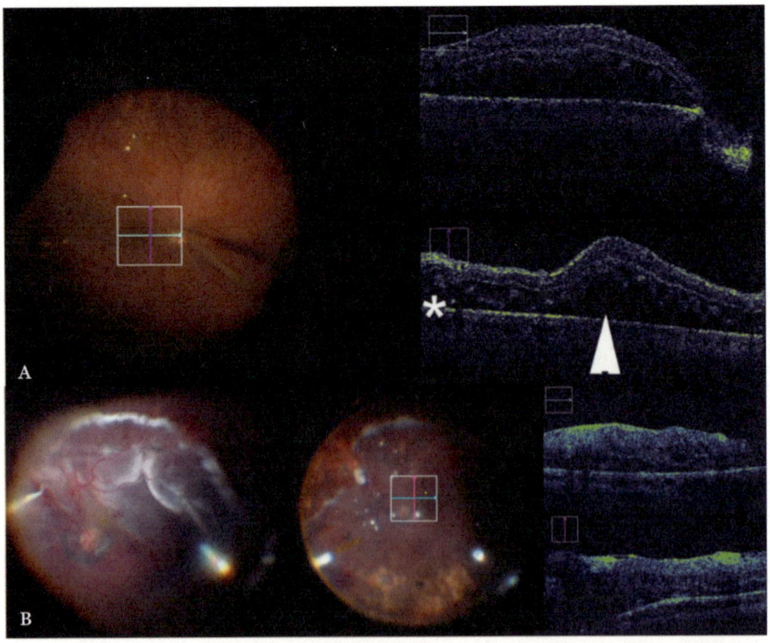

Figure 5.
Color photographs and microscope-integrated optical coherence tomography (MIOCT) scans of retinal detachment surgeries. (A) Real-time horizontal and vertical MIOCT scans during retinal detachment repair under perfluorocarbon liquid evidence the progressive displacement of subretinal fluid (arrowhead) and a discrete subclinical remnant of subretinal fluid under the perfluorocarbon liquid (asterisk) [33]. (B) Complex retinal detachment repair. Color photograph evidences severe vitreoretinal proliferation and subretinal band; endodiathermy has been applied superiorly (left image). Visualization under perfluorocarbon liquid after retinectomy shows a flattened retina (center image). Horizontal and vertical MIOCT scans evidence the reattached retina with scant subclinical subretinal fluid and some residual focal membranes and retinal thickening (right images) [65].

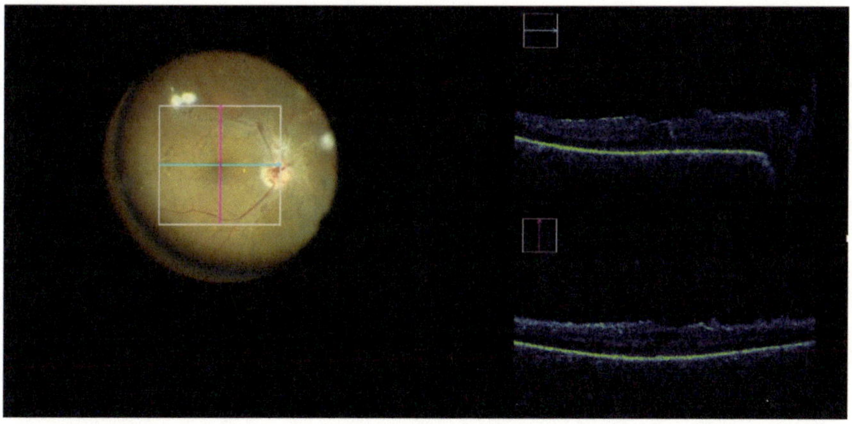

Figure 6.
Macular scan after pars plana vitrectomy in a patient with proliferative diabetic retinopathy. The b-scans evidence minor cystic edema and preserved macular architecture. After image assessment, the surgeon decided not to perform internal limiting membrane peeling.

identification and visualization of the surgical planes to aid membrane dissection, delineate areas of retinal detachment, or topographically localize hemorrhages (e.g., subhyaloid, sub-ILM, or subretinal hemorrhages) [31, 33, 54]. Cases of proliferative diabetic retinopathy with clinically significant macular edema can be optimally assessed to decide if an ILM peeling is needed (**Figure 6**) [55–58]. These clinical circumstances could potentially represent a scenario in which the use of MIOCT can facilitate surgery and enhance outcomes.

2.4 Pediatric retinal surgery

The age and cooperation of the pediatric patients make MIOCT a potentially useful tool to deploy in the examination under general anesthesia, in order to improve the understanding of pathologies such as retinopathy of prematurity (ROP), shaken baby syndrome, or any other vitreoretinal conditions that do not necessarily require VPP, like retinoblastoma [59–62]. Retinoschisis, preretinal structures and membranes, as well as lamellar or full-thickness retinal holes, which were not previously appreciated during an office examination, can be evidenced in ROP or shaken baby syndromes, respectively [59, 62].

2.5 Other vitreoretinal conditions

Chorioretinal biopsy cases could be benefitted by the correct identification of the anatomical layers conforming the surgical plane and differentiation between normal tissue and lesion. The aid of MIOCT can impact on retinal prostheses implantation (e.g., Argus II implants for retinitis pigmentosa), providing precise information of the implant location and allowing a correct positioning [33, 63, 64].

3. Conclusion

The rapid technological evolution of our era has allowed us to consider this potentially powerful field of imaging to further improve retinal surgery. Evidence has demonstrated that MIOCT is feasible and useful in the operating theater, providing valuable information to evaluate the surgical field in real time which can alter surgical decision-making, positively impact on short- and long-term outcomes, and possibly promote the development of new surgical techniques. In the near future, improvements in OCT-compatible surgical instrumentation, feedback systems, and software are warranted to achieve an integration of this technology to our operating theaters.

Conflict of interest

The authors have no commercial or economic conflict of interest to disclose.

Author details

Jesus Hernan Gonzalez-Cortes*, Abraham Olvera-Barrios, Jesus Emiliano Gonzalez-Cantu and Jesus Mohamed-Hamsho

Universidad Autonoma de Nuevo Leon, Ophthalmology Department, Faculty of Medicine and University Hospital "Dr. Jose Eleuterio Gonzalez", Monterrey, Nuevo León, Mexico

*Address all correspondence to: drjesusgzz@gmail.com

References

[1] Barraquer JI. The history of the microscope in ocular surgery. Journal of Microsurgery. 1980;**1**:288-299

[2] Roper-Hall MJ. Microsurgery in ophthalmology. The British Journal of Ophthalmology. 1967;**51**(6):408-414. DOI: 10.1136/bjo.51.6.408

[3] Littmann H. Ein neues Operations-Mikroskop. Klinische Monatsblätter für Augenheilkunde. 1954;**124**:473-476

[4] Harms H, Mackensen G. Augenoperationen unter dem Mikroskop. Tübingen. Verlag. Stuttgart. 1966. Ocular Surgery under the microscope. Year Book Medical Publishers Chicago, 1967

[5] Dekking H. Use of the binocular microscope in eye operations. Archives of Ophthalmology. 1956;**55**:114-117

[6] Keeler CR. 150 years since Babbage's ophthalmoscope. Archives of Ophthalmology. 1997;**115**(11):1456-1457

[7] Parel JM, Machemer R, Aumayr W. A new concept for vitreous surgery. 5. An automated operating microscope. American Journal of Ophthalmology. 1974;**77**(2):161-168. DOI: 10.1016/0002-9394(74)90668-0

[8] Huang D, Swanson EA, Lin CP, et al. Optical coherence tomography. Science. 1991;**254**(5035):1178-1181. DOI: 10.1002/jcp.24872.The

[9] Hee MR, Puliafito CA, Wong C, et al. Optical coherence tomography of macular holes. Ophthalmology. 1995;**102**(5):748-756. DOI: 10.1016/S0161-6420(95)30959-1

[10] Chauhan DS, Marshall J. The interpretation of optical coherence tomography images of the retina. Investigative Ophthalmology and Visual Science. 1999;**40**:2332-2342

[11] Adhi M, Duker JS. Optical coherence tomography-current and future applications. Current Opinion in Ophthalmology. 2013;**24**(3):213-221. DOI: 10.1097/ICU.0b013e32835f8bf8

[12] Chen TC, Cense B, Pierce MC, et al. Spectral domain optical coherence tomography ultra-high speed, ultra-high resolution ophthalmic imaging. Archives of Ophthalmology. 2005;**123**(12):1715-1720. DOI: 10.1001/archopht.123.12.1715

[13] Joshi MM, Trese MT, Capone A. Optical coherence tomography findings in stage 4A retinopathy of prematurity. A theory for visual variability. Ophthalmology. 2006;**13**(4):657-660. DOI: 10.1016/j.ophtha.2006.01.007

[14] Vinekar A, Sivakumar M, Shetty R, et al. A novel technique using spectral-domain optical coherence tomography (Spectralis, SD-OCT+HRA) to image supine non-anaesthetized infants: Utility demonstrated in aggressive posterior retinopathy of prematurity. Eye. 2010;**24**(2):379-382. DOI: 10.1038/eye.2009.313

[15] Dayani PN, Maldonado R, Farsiu S, Toth CA. Intraoperative use of handheld spectral domain optical coherence tomography imaging in macular surgery. Retina. 2009;**29**(10):1457-1468. DOI: 10.1097/IAE.0b013e3181b266bc

[16] Ray R, Baraano DE, Fortun JA, et al. Intraoperative microscope-mounted spectral domain optical coherence tomography for evaluation of retinal anatomy during macular surgery. Ophthalmology. 2011;**118**(11):2212-2217. DOI: 10.1016/j.ophtha.2011.04.012

[17] Ehlers JP, Dupps WJ, Kaiser PK, et al. The prospective intraoperative and perioperative ophthalmic imagiNg with optical coherEncE tomogRaphy

(PIONEER) study: 2-year results. American Journal of Ophthalmology. 2014;**158**(5):999-1007. DOI: 10.1016/j.ajo.2014.07.034

[18] Chavala SH, Farsiu S, Maldonado R, Wallace DK, Freedman SF, Toth CA. Insights into advanced retinopathy of prematurity using handheld spectral domain optical coherence tomography imaging. Ophthalmology. 2009;**116**(12):2448-2456. DOI: 10.1016/j.ophtha.2009.06.003

[19] Maldonado RS, Izatt JA, Sarin N, et al. Optimizing hand-held spectral domain optical coherence tomography imaging for neonates, infants, and children. Investigative Ophthalmology and Visual Science. 2010;**51**(5):2678-2685. DOI: 10.1167/iovs.09-4403

[20] Ehlers JP, Tam T, Kaiser PK, Martin DF, Smith GM, Srivastava SK. Utility of intraoperative optical coherence tomography during vitrectomy surgery for vitreomacular traction syndrome. Retina. 2014;**34**(7):1341-1346. DOI: 10.1097/IAE.0000000000000123

[21] Branchini LA, Gurley K, Duker JS, Reichel E. Use of handheld intraoperative spectral-domain optical coherence tomography in a variety of vitreoretinal diseases. Ophthalmic Surgery, Lasers and Imaging Retina. 2016;**47**(1):49-54. DOI: 10.3928/23258160-20151214-07

[22] Ehlers JP, Kernstine K, Farsiu S, Sarin N, Maldonado R, Toth CA. Analysis of pars plana vitrectomy for optic pit-related maculopathy with intraoperative optical coherence tomography: A possible connection with the vitreous cavity. Archives of Ophthalmology. 2011;**129**(11):1483-1486. DOI: 10.1001/archophthalmol.2011.316

[23] Binder S, Falkner-Radler CI, Hauger C, Matz H, Glittenberg C. Feasibility of intrasurgical spectral-domain optical coherence tomography. Retina. 2011;**31**(7):1332-1336. DOI: 10.1097/IAE.0b013e3182019c18

[24] Ehlers JP, Ohr MP, Kaiser PK, Srivastava SK. Novel microarchitectural dynamics in rhegmatogenous retinal detachments identified with intraoperative optical coherence tomography. Retina. 2013;**33**(7):1428-1434. DOI: 10.1097/IAE.0b013e31828396b7

[25] Boppart SA, Bouma BE, Pitris C, et al. Intraoperative assessment of microsurgery with three-dimensional optical coherence tomography. Radiology. 1998;**208**(1):81-86. DOI: 10.1148/radiology.208.1.9646796

[26] Lankenau E, Klinger D, Winter C, et al. Combining optical coherence tomography (OCT) with an operating microscope. Advances in Medical Engineering. 2007;**114**:343-348. DOI: 10.1007/978-3-540-68764-1_57

[27] Tao YK, Ehlers JP, Toth CA, Izatt JA. Intraoperative spectral domain optical coherence tomography for vitreoretinal surgery. Optics Letters. 2010;**35**(20):3315-3317. DOI: 10.1364/OL.35.003315

[28] Geerling G, Müller M, Winter C, et al. Intraoperative 2-dimensional optical coherence tomography as a new tool for anterior segment surgery. Archives of Ophthalmology. 2005;**123**(2):253-257. DOI: 10.1001/archopht.123.2.253

[29] Steven P, Le Blanc C, Velten K, et al. Optimizing descemet membrane endothelial keratoplasty using intraoperative optical coherence tomography. JAMA Ophthalmology. 2013;**131**(9):1135-1142. DOI: 10.1001/jamaophthalmol.2013.4672

[30] Ehlers JP, Kaiser PK, Srivastava SK. Intraoperative optical coherence tomography using the RESCAN 700: Preliminary results from the DISCOVER study. The British Journal of

Ophthalmology. 2014;**98**(10):1329-1332. DOI: 10.1136/bjophthalmol-2014-305294

[31] Ehlers JP, Goshe J, Dupps WJ, et al. Determination of feasibility and utility of microscope-integrated optical coherence tomography during ophthalmic surgery: The DISCOVER study RESCAN results. JAMA Ophthalmology. 2015;**133**(10):1124-1132. DOI: 10.1001/jamaophthalmol.2015.2376

[32] Cost B, Goshe JM, Srivastava S, Ehlers JP. Intraoperative optical coherence tomography-assisted descemet membrane endothelial keratoplasty in the DISCOVER study. American Journal of Ophthalmology. 2015;**160**(3):430-437. DOI: 10.1016/j.ajo.2015.05.020

[33] Ehlers JP, Modi YS, Pecen PE, et al. The DISCOVER study 3-year results: Feasibility and usefulness of microscope-integrated intraoperative OCT during ophthalmic surgery. Ophthalmology. 2018;**125**(7):1014-1027. DOI: 10.1016/j.ophtha.2017.12.037

[34] Khan M, Srivastava SK, Reese JL, Shwani Z, Ehlers JP. Intraoperative OCT-assisted surgery for proliferative diabetic retinopathy in the DISCOVER study. Ophthalmology Retina. 2018;**2**(5):411-417. DOI: 10.1016/j.oret.2017.08.020

[35] Falkner-Radler CI, Glittenberg C, Gabriel M, Binder S. Intrasurgical microscopeintegrated spectral domain optical coherence tomography-assisted membrane peeling. Retina. 2015;**35**(10):2100-2106. DOI: 10.1097/IAE.0000000000000596

[36] Hahn P, Migacz J, O'Connell R, et al. Preclinical evaluation and intraoperative human retinal imaging with a high-resolution microscope-integrated spectral domain optical coherence tomography device. Retina. 2013;**33**(7):1328-1337. DOI: 10.1097/IAE.0b013e3182831293

[37] Leisser C, Hackl C, Hirnschall N, et al. Visualizing macular structures during membrane peeling surgery with an intraoperative spectral-domain optical coherence tomography device. Ophthalmic Surgery, Lasers and Imaging Retina. 2016;**47**(4):328-332. DOI: 10.3928/23258160-20160324-04

[38] Pfau M, Michels S, Binder S, Becker MD. Clinical experience with the first commercially available intraoperative optical coherence tomography system. Ophthalmic Surgery, Lasers and Imaging Retina. 2015;**46**(10):1001-1008. DOI: 10.3928/23258160-20151027-03

[39] Ramírez-Estudillo JA, Sánchez-Ramos JA, Pérez-Montaño CR, González-Cortés JH. Utilidad transquirúrgica de la tomografía de coherencia óptica en cirugía vítreo-retiniana. Cirugía y Cirujanos. 2017;**85**(1):21-26. DOI: 10.1016/j.circir.2016.04.002

[40] Ehlers JP, Khan M, Petkovsek D, et al. Outcomes of intraoperative OCT–assisted epiretinal membrane surgery from the PIONEER study. Ophthalmology Retina. 2018;**2**(4):263-267. DOI: 10.1016/j.oret.2017.05.006

[41] Ehlers JP, Han J, Petkovsek D, Kaiser PK, Singh RP, Srivastava SK. Membrane peeling-induced retinal alterations on intraoperative OCT in vitreomacular interface disorders from the PIONEER study. Investigative Ophthalmology and Visual Science. 2015;**56**(12):7324-7330. DOI: 10.1167/iovs.15-17526

[42] Nam DH, Desouza PJ, Hahn P, et al. Intraoperative spectral domain optical coherence tomography imaging after internal limiting membrane peeling in idiopathic epiretinal membrane with connecting strands. Retina. 2015;**35**(8):1622-1630. DOI: 10.1097/IAE.0000000000000534

[43] Farah ME, Maia M, Penha FM, Rodrigues EB. The use of vital dyes during vitreoretinal surgery-chromovitrectomy. Developments in Ophthalmology. 2015;**55**:365-375. DOI: 10.1159/000438963

[44] Salvetti AP, Patrício MI, Barnard AR, Orlans HO, Hickey DG, MacLaren RE. Impact of vital dyes on cell viability and transduction efficiency of AAV vectors used in retinal gene therapy surgery: An in vitro and In vivo analysis. Translational Vision Science & Technology. 2017;**6**(4):4. DOI: 10.1167/tvst.6.4.4

[45] Penha FM, Pons M, Costa Ede P, et al. Effect of vital dyes on retinal pigmented epithelial cell viability and apoptosis: Implications for chromovitrectomy. Ophthalmologica. 2013;**230**(2):41-50. DOI: 10.1159/000354251

[46] Gonzalez-Cortes JH, Estudillo AR, Sanchez-Ramos JA, Bages-Rousselon Y, Fernandez-Mar M, Mohamed-Hamsho J. Anatomical changes of full-thickness macular hole documented by microscope-integrated spectral-domain optical coherence tomography. Ophthalmic Surgery, Lasers and Imaging Retina. 2018;**49**(9):e105-e111. DOI: 10.3928/23258160-20180907-17

[47] Ehlers JP, Xu D, Kaiser PK, Singh RP, Srivastava SK. Intrasurgical dynamics of macular hole surgery: An assessment of surgery-induced ultrastructural alterations with intraoperative optical coherence tomography. Retina. 2014;**34**(2):213-221. DOI: 10.1097/IAE.0b013e318297daf3

[48] Hahn P, Migacz J, O'Connell R, Izatt JA, Toth CA. Unprocessed real-time imaging of vitreoretinal surgical maneuvers using a microscope-integrated spectral-domain optical coherence tomography system. Graefe's Archive for Clinical and Experimental Ophthalmology. 2013;**251**(1):213-220. DOI: 10.1007/s00417-012-2052-2

[49] Hahn P, Carrasco-Zevallos O, Cunefare D, et al. Intrasurgical human retinal imaging with manual instrument tracking using a microscope-integrated spectral-domain optical coherence tomography device. Translational Vision Science & Technology. 2015;**4**(4):1. DOI: 10.1167/tvst.4.4.1

[50] Xu D, Yuan A, Kaiser PK, et al. A novel segmentation algorithm for volumetric analysis of macular hole boundaries identified with optical coherence tomography. Investigative Ophthalmology and Visual Science. 2013;**54**:163-169. DOI: 10.1167/iovs.12-10246

[51] Ehlers JP, Itoh Y, Xu LT, Kaiser PK, Singh RP, Srivastava SK. Factors associated with persistent subfoveal fluid and complete macular hole closure in the PIONEER study. Investigative Ophthalmology and Visual Science. 2015;**56**(2):1141-1146. DOI: 10.1167/iovs.14-15765

[52] Itoh Y, Vasanji A, Ehlers JP. Volumetric ellipsoid zone mapping for enhanced visualisation of outer retinal integrity with optical coherence tomography. The British Journal of Ophthalmology. 2016;**100**(3):295-299. DOI: 10.1136/bjophthalmol-2015-307105

[53] Smith AG, Cost BM, Ehlers JP, Intraoperative OCT-assisted subretinal perfuorocarbon liquid removal in the DISCOVER study. Ophthalmic Surely, Lasers and Imaging Retina. 2015;**49**(9):964-966. DOI: 10.3928/23258160-20151008-10

[54] Oellers P, Mahmoud TH. Surgery for proliferative diabetic retinopathy: New tips and tricks. Journal of Ophthalmic and Vision Research. 2016;**11**(1):93-99. DOI: 10.4103/2008-322X.180697

[55] Bhagat N, Grigorian RA, Tutela A, Zarbin MA. Diabetic macular edema: Pathogenesis and treatment. Survey of Ophthalmology. 2009;**54**(1):1-32. DOI: 10.1016/j.survophthal.2008.10.001

[56] Dehghan MH, Salehipour M, Naghib J, Babaeian M, Karimi S, Yaseri M. Pars plana vitrectomy with internal limiting membrane peeling for refractory diffuse diabetic macular edema. Journal of Ophthalmic and Vision Research. 2010;**5**(3):162-167. DOI: 10.1097/IAE.0b013e31816102f2

[57] Patel JI, Hykin PG, Schadt M, Luong VY, Fitzke F, Gregor ZJ. Pars plana vitrectomy with and without peeling of the inner limiting membrane for diabetic macular edema. Retina. 2006;**26**(1):5-13. DOI: 10.1097/00006982-200601000-00002

[58] Gandorfer A, Messmer EM, Ulbig MW, Kampik A. Resolution of diabetic macular edema after surgical removal of the posterior hyaloid and the inner limiting membrane. Retina. 2000;**20**(2):126-133. DOI: 10.1097/00006982-200002000-00004

[59] Rachitskaya AV, Yuan A, Marino MJ, Reese J, Ehlers JP. Intraoperative OCT imaging of the Argus II retinal prosthesis system. Ophthalmic Surgery, Lasers and Imaging Retina. 2016;**47**(11):999-1003. DOI: 10.3928/23258160-20161031-03

[60] Browne AW, Ehlers JP, Sharma S, Srivastava SK. Intraoperative optical coherence tomography-assisted chorioretinal biopsy in the DISCOVER study. Retina. 2017;**37**(11):2183-2187. DOI: 10.1097/IAE.0000000000001522

[61] Seider MI, Tran-Viet D, Toth CA. Macular pseudo-hole in shaken baby syndrome: Underscoring the utility of optical coherence tomography under anesthesia. Retinal Cases and Brief Reports. 2016;**10**(3):283-285. DOI: 10.1097/ICB.0000000000000251

[62] Rootman DB, Gonzalez E, Mallipatna A, et al. Hand-held high-resolution spectral domain optical coherence tomography in retinoblastoma: Clinical and morphologic considerations. The British Journal of Ophthalmology. 2013;**97**(1):59-65. DOI: 10.1136/bjophthalmol-2012-302133

[63] Cao C, Markovitz M, Ferenczy S, Shields CL. Hand-held spectral-domain optical coherence tomography of small macular retinoblastoma in infants before and after chemotherapy. Journal of Pediatric Ophthalmology and Strabismus. 2014;**51**(4):230-234. DOI: 10.3928/01913913-20140603-01

[64] Campbell JP, Nudleman E, Yang J, et al. Handheld optical coherence tomography angiography and ultra-wide-field optical coherence tomography in retinopathy of prematurity. JAMA Ophthalmology. 2017;**135**(9):977-981. DOI: 10.1001/jamaophthalmol.2017.2481

[65] Ehlers JP, Uchida A, Srivastava SK. The integrative surgical theater: Combining intraoperative optical coherence tomography and 3D digital visualization for Vitreoretinal surgery in THE DISCOVER study. Retina. 2018;**38**(Suppl 1):S88-S96. DOI: 10.1097/IAE.0000000000001999

Section 3

Posterior Eye Segment Diagnostic Methods

Chapter 4

Wide-Field Retinal Imaging in Adults and Children

Mustafa Değer Bilgeç, Nazmiye Erol and Seyhan Topbaş

Abstract

Wide-field retinal imaging has become an important standard of care imaging modality in many retinal disorders both in adults and children. The recently developed wide-field retinal imaging systems enable approximately 200° imaging of retina. In this chapter, we would like to review the use of wide-field retinal imaging in disorders such as retinal vascular diseases, uveal and retinal inflammatory diseases, intraocular tumors, peripheral retinal pathologies, and retinal disorders in children such as retinopathy of prematurity, familial exudative vitreoretinopathy, and Coats' disease. Also, we would like to address the rapidly expanding role of peripheral retinal imaging in treating systemic diseases. The use of wide-field imaging technologies in screening, diagnosis, treatment, and documentation of retinal pathologies and the new information provided by wide-field angiography for retinal vascular diseases and macular problems will be discussed.

Keywords: retinal imaging, wide-field, ultra-wide-field, wide-angle, fluorescein angiography, optomap, scanning laser ophthalmoscope

1. Introduction

Wide-field retinal imaging gives the opportunity to simultaneously visualize the central and peripheral retina in a single session. Older wide-field retinal imaging systems had significant downsides such as the requirement of a contact lens and a clear ocular media [1]. Acquiring images from the far peripheral retina was difficult, requiring a skilled technician and demanded difficult tasks from the patient such as performing extreme gazes. Systems that utilized image montaging could only capture up to 75° of the retina and were disadvantaged due to frequent montage errors [1–3]. New-generation devices were able to obtain up to 140° at one session [1–3].

The Optos Optomap Panoramic 200A imaging system (Optos® camera,Optos PLC, Dunfermline, UK) revolutionized wide-field retinal imaging by increasing the field of view to 200° [4]. This system implements a scanning laser ophthalmoscope technology with an ellipsoid mirror and covers approximately 82% of the retina in a single image by forming a virtual scanning head within the patient's eye [1]. Compared with conventional digital imaging systems, ultra-wide-field fluorescein angiography (UWFA) using the Optos system captures twice as much retinal area [5]. Heidelberg (Heidelberg Engineering, Germany) introduced a noncontact lens that attaches to the Heidelberg Spectralis and Retinal Angiography systems allowing ultra-wide-field photography and angiography [6].

Endowed with high resolution and multimodal capabilities, ultra-wide-field imaging is destined to become the standard-of-care in retinal imaging. These

Confocal scanning laser ophthalmoscope(CSLO)-based systems	Optos, Heidelberg
Optics-based systems	RetCam, Panoret 1000
Contact lens-based systems	Staurenghi, Rodenstock lens

Table 1.
Classification of wide-field devices according to their working principles.

devices have also found their place in research applications and have the potential to be utilized in telemedicine [7]. Wide-angle imaging systems using different systems are summarized in **Table 1**.

2. The history and evolution of retinal imaging

Hermann von Helmholtz was the founder of the first direct ophthalmoscope in 1851 [8]. The first available fundus camera, produced by Carl Zeiss in 1955, had a 20° field of vision. Development of fluorescein angiography (FA) in 1961 brought another format to retinal imaging [9]. The first camera that was able to visualize beyond the equator was developed by Oleg Pomerantzeff in 1977 and this device could image 148° of the retinal area. A disadvantage of this modality was the requirement of a contact lens and transscleral illumination [10]. In the meantime, montage methods had been developed to image the peripheral retina such as the 75° views compiled for the ETDRS seven-standard fields [1, 3]. A further development in the wide-field imaging systems was the introduction of RetCam (Clarity Medical Systems, Inc., Pleasanton, CA, USA) by Bert Messie in 1997 which was able to image up to 130°. This device which brought significant convenience in pediatric retinal imaging was quickly popularized [9]. The main disadvantage of this device is its optical method of illumination, necessitating a clear media. In 2003, Medibell introduced the Panoret-1000 (Medibell Medical Vision Technologies, Inc., Haifa, Israel), incorporating a non-mydriatic camera which could image up to 100° of the retina. However, this technique was technically demanding as it required technicians for image acquisition. In general, although it was able to capture high-resolution images of the retina, it did not perform well in dark pigmented fundus due to decreased transscleral illumination [9, 11]. A milestone in wide-field retinal imaging systems was the development of Optos in 2005 (Optos® camera,Optos PLC, Dunfermline, UK) which, by utilizing an ellipsoidal mirror, was capable of capturing up to 200° of the internal viewing angle of the retina [4]. Both UWFA and fundus autofluorescence are available. Furthermore, this UWFA system allowed better detection of peripheral capillary non-perfusion. An indocyanine green (ICG) angiography upgrade was also recently made available [6, 9]. In 2005, Giovanni Staurenghi developed the handheld Staurenghi 230 SLO Retina Lens (Ocular Staurenghi 230 SLO Retina Lens; Ocular Instrument Inc., Bellevue, WA, USA) which was later incorporated into a confocal scanning laser ophthalmoscopy system by Heidelberg. Addition of this lens increased the original field of view of Heidelberg Retinal Angiography (HRA) Spectralis system from 100° to 150° of the retina [12].

In summary, apart from Optos, other notable systems for wide-field imaging include the Pomerantzeff Camera/Equator-plus, Panoret-1000, the Staurenghi lens, HRA Spectralis and RetCam 3 system [11–15]. Each of the former devices has its specific inherent limitations such as the requirement of a contact lens, illumination difficulties, low resolution, optical aberrations limiting angiographic view, incapability to obtain ultra-wide-field retinal images, and absence of ultra-wide-field autofluorescence imaging. Although the montage method using standard fundus photography is also able to obtain wide-angle images of the retina, the final assembled image may not be synchronous as none of the images have been captured simultaneously [16].

3. Advantages of modern digital wide-field imaging systems

- Enhanced resolution
- Faster image processing time
- Faster image acquisition
- Ease of image duplication and manipulation
- Possibility of image transmission via electronic route
- Better acquisition in eyes with hazy ocular media (such as cataract) than a traditional fundus camera
- Simultaneous imaging of central and peripheral retina [17].

4. Confocal scanning laser ophthalmoscopy imaging (CSLO) systems

CSLO systems use laser light to illuminate the retina, instead of bright flashes of light. This reduces scatter of light in images acquired. Two different wavelengths of laser are used (532 nm-green, 633 nm-red). Green laser provides more detailed information about the superficial layers of the retina and the retinal vessels. Red laser (633 nm) owing to a longer wavelength gives more detailed information about deep retinal layers and choroid. Images can be evaluated separately or a composite photo image is acquired [18].

5. Multimodal imaging with digital wide-field systems

A great advantage offered by many of the present WFI and UWFI systems is the possibility of simultaneous acquisition of fundus fluorescein angiography (FA), indocyanine angiography (ICGA), red-free photography, fundus photography, fundus autofluorescence (FAF), including blue-light fundus autofluorescence (BAF), infrared autofluorescence (IRAF) or green-light fundus autofluorescence (GAF). The main features of commercially available WFI systems are summarized in **Table 2**.

	Platforms/devices	Type of lens system	Principle	Field of view	Available application
WFI	Heidelberg Spectralis	Non-contact	SD-OCT with CSLO	55°(105°with HRA2)	FFA, ICGA, FAF(BAF and IRAF)
		Contact	SD-OCT with CSLO using Staurenghi Lens	150°	FFA,ICGA, FAF(BAF and IRAF)

	Platforms/devices	Type of lens system	Principle	Field of view	Available application
	RetCam 3	Contact	Optical light source to obtain high resolution	130°	FFA, ICGA
UWFI	Optos	Non-contact	CSLO-based	200	FFA,FAF (GAF,IRAF),ICGA

Table 2.
The main features of commercially available WFI systems.

6. Wide-field fundus autofluorescence (FAF) imaging

Autofluorescence is based on the excitation of fluorophores within the retina. The main fluorophore is lipofuscin, found in the retinal pigment epithelial cells [19]. For some diseases, autofluorescence provides valuable information in the differential diagnosis. An ultra-wide-field scanning laser ophthalmoscope with FAF capability was recently introduced. The importance of peripheral retinal evaluation was highlighted in reports showing distinct peripheral FAF changes in diseases that were previously assumed to be isolated to macula [20]. Wide-field FAF imaging

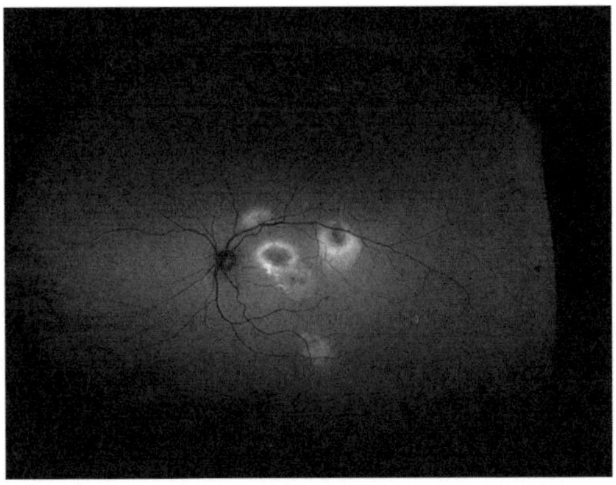

Figure 1.
Typical FAF appearance of multifocal central serious chorioretinopathy. Hyperfluorescent areas are indicative of chronic subretinal fluid and secondary RPE changes.

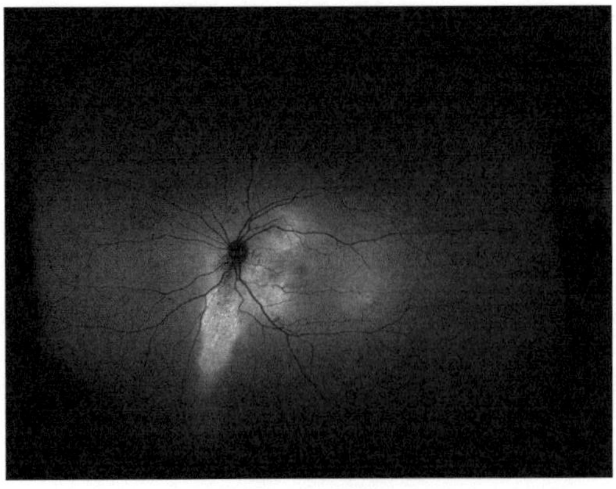

Figure 2.
FAF shows a hyper-autofluorescent gravitational tract in chronic central serous chorioretinopathy.

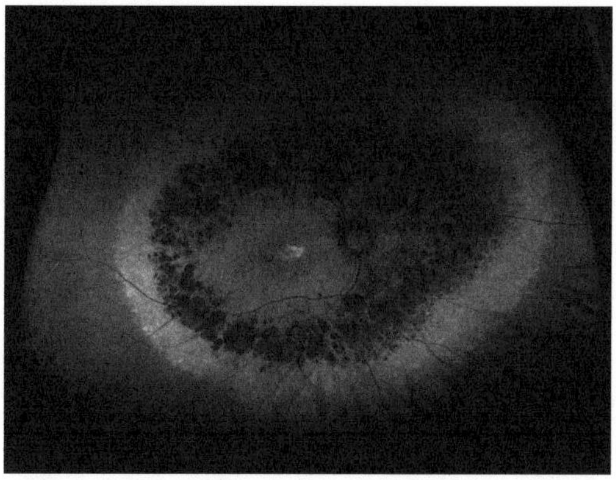

Figure 3.
FAF image of a patient with retinitis pigmentosa showing annular hypo and hyper autofluorescent areas.

provides valuable information in pathologies such as AMD, posterior uveitis, and choroidal melanoma [21]. Wide-field imaging also provides valuable clinical data in central serous chorioretinopathy [22] (**Figures 1–3**).

7. Applications of wide-field imaging in clinical practice

7.1 Healthy eyes

In order to evaluate the pathological angiography findings in various diseases, first of all, it is necessary to evaluate the normal retinal findings in wide-field angiography.[23, 24] Perfused vascular border distance decreases after 60 years of age in all quadrants [24]. Normal peripheral retinas infrequently show granular background fluorescence [23]. **Figure 4** shows wide-field images of healthy eyes.

7.2 Diabetic retinopathy

Vascular abnormalities in diabetic retinopathy, particularly non-perfusion, occur in the peripheral retina; therefore, evaluation of the retinal periphery is of vital importance [25]. With the advent of wide-field imaging systems in recent years, it is possible to evaluate peripheral retina which cannot be visualized by conventional imaging systems in diabetic patients. Peripheral avascular areas, neovascularization, and vascular leakages are evaluated. UWFA was found superior to simulated seven-standard field images in a previous study not only in terms of the visualized total retinal area (3.2 times) but also in terms of the total area of retinal non-perfusion (3.9 times), neovascularization (1.9 times), and panretinal photocoagulation (3.8 times) [26]. Moreover, this study has demonstrated that the seven-standard field image technique has failed to identify positive findings that were present in UWFA in 10% of the patients [26]. Detecting peripheral retinal ischemia is essential as studies have shown that peripheral ischemia may precede diabetic macular edema [27, 28]. In patients with retinal ischemia, macular edema was 3.75 times more than those without ischemia [28]. Patients with diabetic retinopathy with large ischemic areas had more treatment-resistant macular edema [27]. It is stated that ultra-wide-field imaging may provide some additional data in the diagnosis because it contains a larger area [29–32]. **Figure 5** shows UWFA image of a diabetic patient with marked peripheral ischemia.

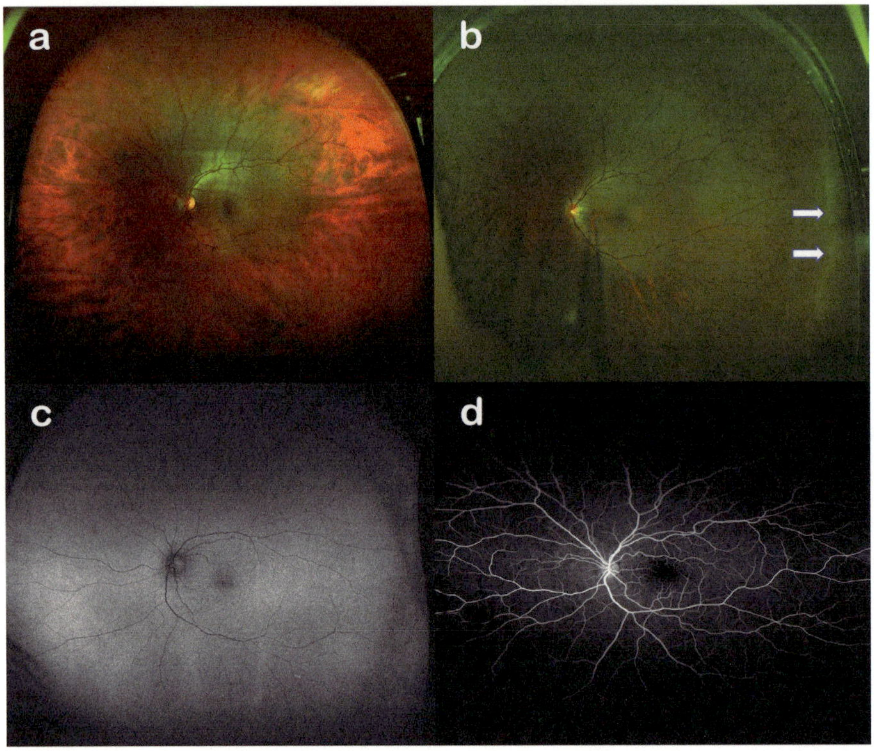

Figure 4.
Various wide-field images in different adults with healthy eyes. Composite color photo (a), pars plana view at temporal gaze (white arrows) (b), normal FAF image (c), and normal FA image (d).

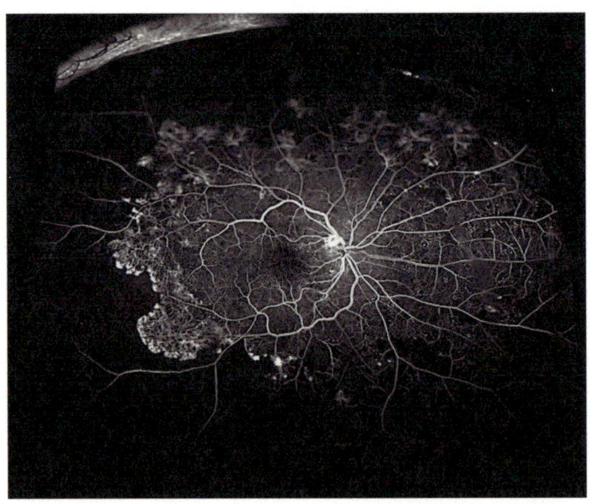

Figure 5.
UWFA image of a patient with diabetic retinopathy showing marked peripheral ischemia, patches of neovascularization at disc and elsewhere.

7.3 Retinal vascular occlusions

7.3.1 Branch retinal vein occlusions

Branch retinal vein occlusion (BRVO) is a significant cause of vision loss and is the second most common retinal vascular disease after diabetic retinopathy. BRVO can be categorized as ischemic or non-ischemic [33]. Wide-field FA can be used to identify vascular abnormalities, peripheral capillary non-perfusion, and neovascularization [34, 35]. Capillary non-perfusion on wide-field angiography heralds the development of macular edema in patients with BRVO [36]. Increased production of VEGF has been proposed to cause macular edema by increasing capillary permeability [36]. **Figure 6** shows UWFA image of a patient with BRVO.

7.3.2 Central retinal vein occlusions

Central retinal vein occlusion (CRVO) is a relatively less frequent cause of vision loss than BRVO. CRVO is classified into ischemic and non-ischemic types depending on the extent of retinal ischemia. As the detection of the extent of retinal ischemia is crucial in prognostication, peripheral retinal imaging is of significant value. Conventional FA systems may be limited in peripheral retinal assessment compared to UWFA. As such, considering that ischemic CRVO is, by definition, the presence of non-perfusion greater than 10 disc diameters, UWFA may be more efficient than conventional FA in differentiating ischemic from non-ischemic CRVOs [37]. Furthermore, wide-field FA allows detection of a greater area of overall non-perfusion enabling earlier and targeted laser photocoagulation [37–39]. In view of these considerations, UWFA is anticipated to improve the management of CRVO. **Figure 7** shows a wide-field fundus photography and UWFA of a patient with CRVO in the acute phase.

7.4 Choroidal lesions including tumors

Wide-field imaging systems ease the evaluation and follow-up of peripheral temporal lesions [40]. SLO images can be distinguished as malignant or benign lesions. Typically, malignant lesions appear dark with a red laser, but appear bright with a green laser [41]. Wide-field fundus imaging may allow documentation of growth of a choroidal tumor and associated serous retinal detachment [42]. **Figures 8** and **9** show two different choroidal tumors imaged by ultra-wide-field imaging system.

7.5 Retinal detachment

Wide-field imaging may be used to supplement fundus examination for characterizing and documenting retinal detachments [7, 43]. Use of wide-field systems in the diagnosis and evaluation of retinal detachments is, however, controversial. The gold

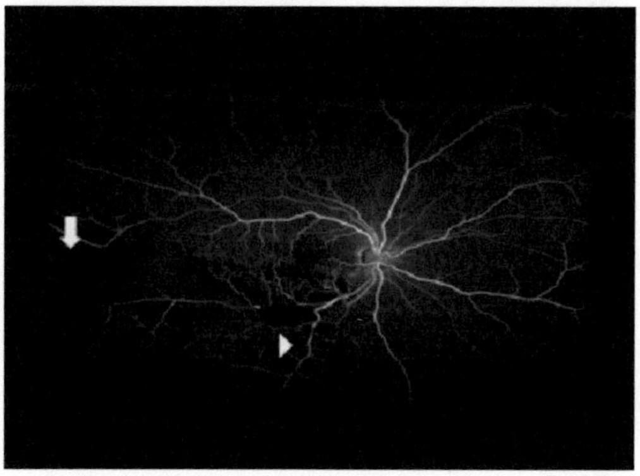

Figure 6.
UWFA image of the inferior temporal region in a patient with BRVO showing a delineated area of peripheral ischemia (arrow) and areas of blocked fluorescence due to hemorrhage (arrow head).

standard in diagnosing retinal detachment remains a dilated binocular indirect examination with scleral depression. **Figure 10** shows a patient with retinal detachment.

7.6 Age-related macular degeneration (AMD)

Detection of peripheral autofluorescence is a potential area of research and its significance is currently being investigated in different studies [44, 45]. In a previous study, peripheral FAF abnormalities were found to be 68.9% and several distinct FAF patterns were identified: granular (46.2%), spotted (34.0%), and nummular (18.1%). An abnormal FAF pattern was observed more frequently in neovascular compared to non-neovascular AMD or normal eyes, but the clinical

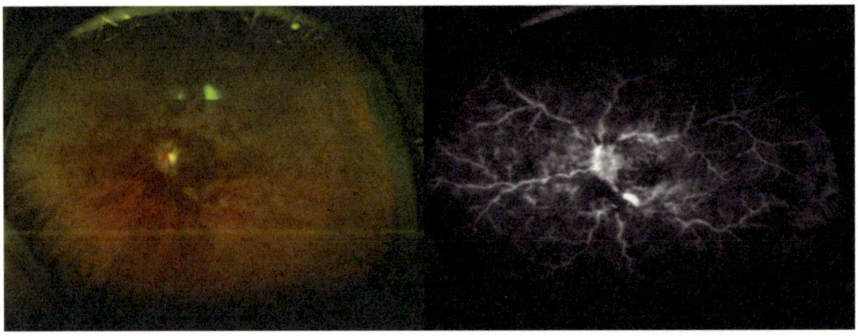

Figure 7.
Wide-field fundus photograph and UWFA image of the left eye of a patient with CRVO illustrating widespread retinal hemorrhage and disc staining. Peripheral ischemia in this patient may have been missed by conventional FA due to limited field of view.

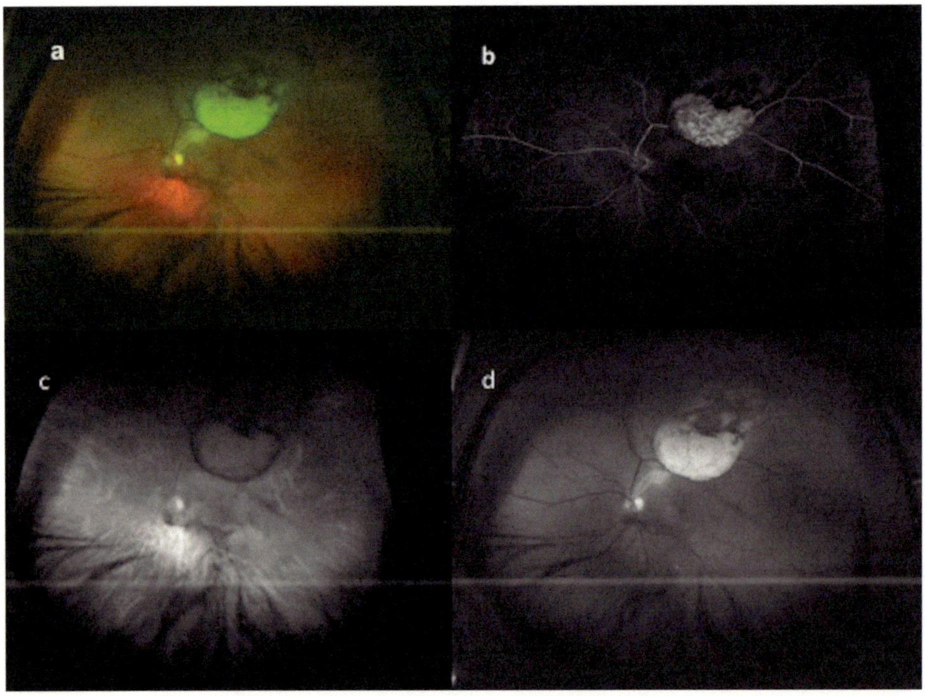

Figure 8.
A case of choroidal malignant melanoma, composite photograph (a), UWFA (b), red laser (c), and green laser/red-free (d) images.

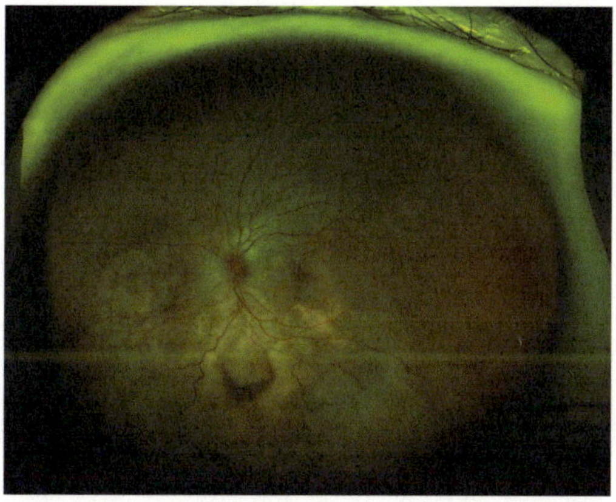

Figure 9.
Wide-field fundus photograph of a choroidal metastatic tumor with exudative retinal detachment in a patient with lung cancer.

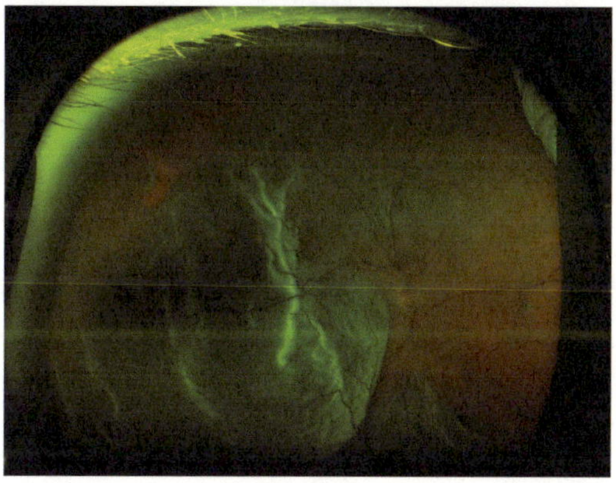

Figure 10.
Macula-off retinal detachment with a horse-shoe tear at 10 o'clock.

significance of these findings is, at present, uncertain [45]. **Figure 11** shows various peripheral FAF abnormalities in different AMD patients.

7.7 Pediatric retinal diseases

Wide-field imaging of retinopathy of prematurity (ROP) is usually performed using RetCam technology. Optos test is performed more often in older children to document the late sequelae of ROP. Even if it seems difficult, Optos imaging of newborns with ROP can also be performed using the "flying baby" position [46]. Wide-field imaging for telemedicine-based screening of ROP has recently gained popularity [47]. RetCam can be used immediately after laser treatment to identify untreated areas in ROP cases [48]. The RetCam technology is also useful in the diagnosis and follow-up of retinoblastoma. UWF imaging with Optos has been shown to be useful in the diagnosis of Coats' disease. Wide-field imaging is critical for the detection of areas of non-perfusion and telangiectasias, in addition image-guided targeted panretinal photocoagulation to these areas [49, 50]. Familial exudative vitreoretinopathy (FEVR) is a condition of abnormal vascularization of the retinal periphery. UWFA has also been employed to conceptualize an updated version of FEVR classification [51]. **Figures 12–15** show images of pediatric patients with different retinal diseases.

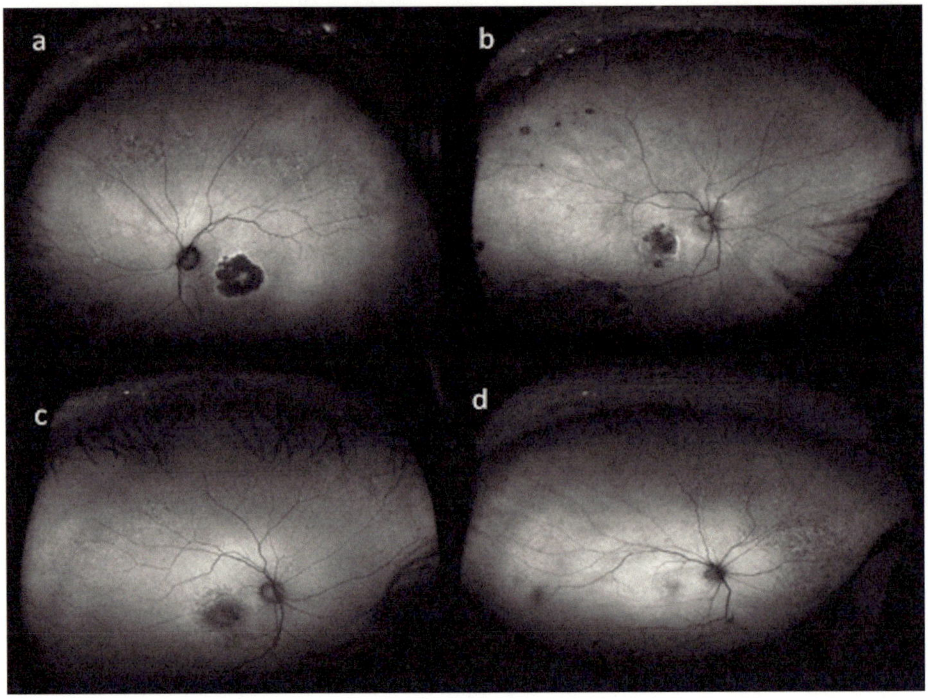

Figure 11.
Various peripheral FAF abnormalities in different AMD patients. Hypo-autofluorescent lesions with hyper-autofluorescent borders (a), nummular hypo-autofluorescent lesions (b), hyper-autofluorescent lesions (c), and hypo-autofluorescent lesions (d) at peripheral retina.

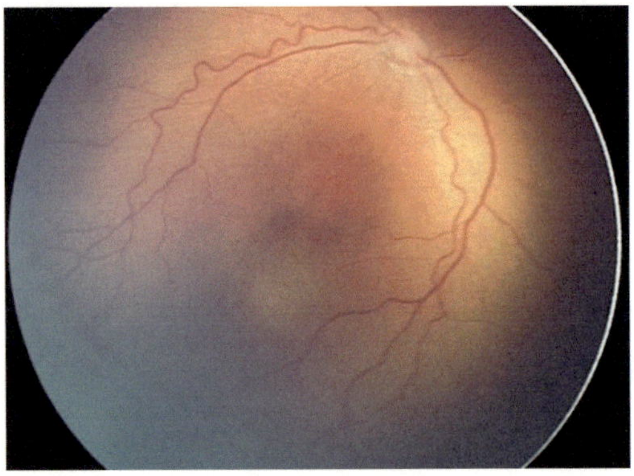

Figure 12.
Color fundus photograph reveals zone II, stage 2 retinopathy of prematurity with plus disease (from RetCam).

7.8 Uveitis

UWFA is useful in evaluating disease severity, progression, and treatment response in intermediate or posterior uveitis [52]. The UWFA showed a view of capillary dropout and leakage in the peripheral retina. This was first demonstrated in two case series of patients with retinal vasculitis imaged with UWFA [53, 54]. In a study about Behçet retinal vasculitis, it was found that UWFA detected active vasculitis not otherwise detectable in 84.8% of eyes [55]. Multimodal UWF imaging will likely assume a more prominent role in the diagnosis and follow-up of patients with retinal vasculitis and posterior uveitis [7]. **Figures 16–18** show images of different uveitis patients in wide-field imaging.

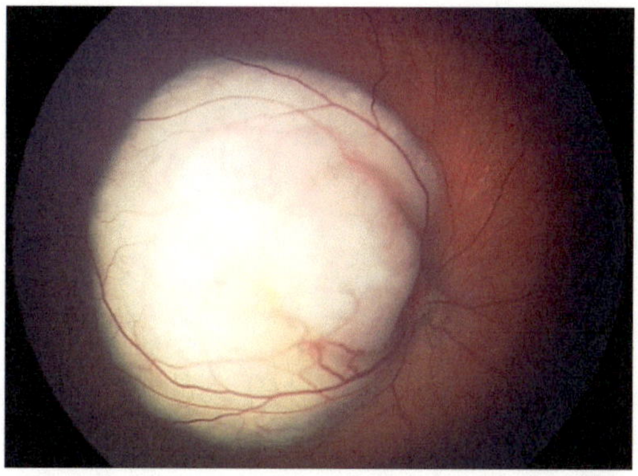

Figure 13.
A RetCam image of a retinoblastoma case showing a large retinal mass encompassing the retinal arcuates.

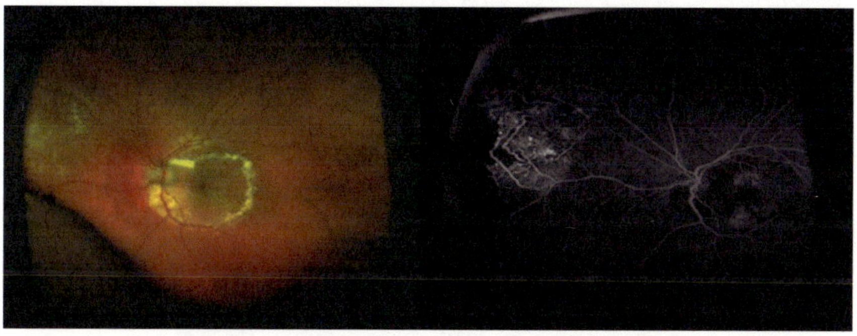

Figure 14.
Wide-field fundus photograph (left panel) of a patient with Coats' disease showing macular circinate exudates, telangiectatic vessels in the upper nasal retina. UWFA image (right panel) of the same patient showing telangiectatic vessels and peripheral non-perfusion.

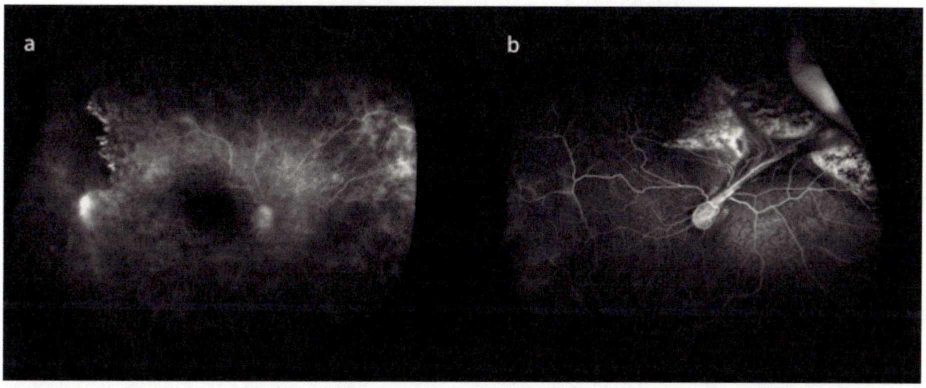

Figure 15.
UWFA image of the right (a) and left eye (b) of a patient with FEVR. Marked peripheral retinal non-perfusion and NVE (a) and severe macular dragging due to falciform retinal fold (b) is noted.

7.9 Miscellaneous diseases

UWFA shows peripheral perfusion abnormalities not previously recognized in myopic eyes. Retinal vasculature in the peripheral retina is significantly altered in eyes with axial myopia. This may be associated to a mechanical stretching [56].

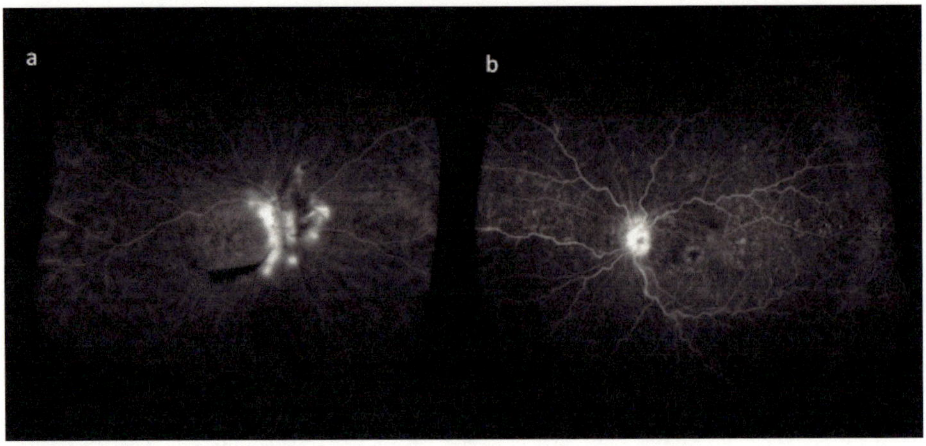

Figure 16.
Diffuse vasculitic leakage and neovascularization at disc (NVD) in a case with Behçet's disease (a) and diffuse vasculitic leakage and macular edema in a patient with idiopathic retinal vasculitis (b).

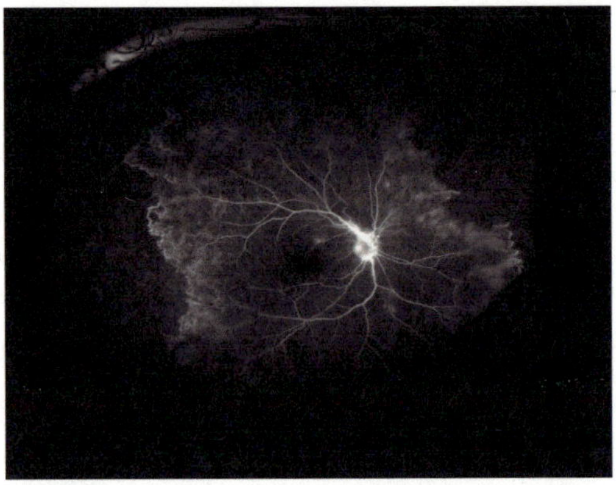

Figure 17.
Wide-field fundus photograph and UWFA image of the left eye of a patient with Eales disease. Peripheral ischemia in the nasal and temporal quadrants accompanied by collateral formation and NVD.

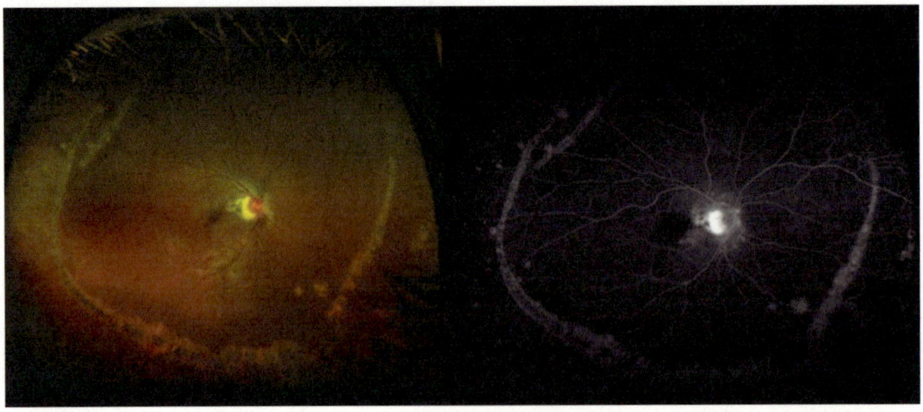

Figure 18.
Wide-field fundus photograph and UWFA images of the right eye showing mid-peripheral linear lesions (Schlaegel lines) and secondary peripapillary CNV. This patient was diagnosed with multifocal choroiditis.

UWFI has shown a significant association between Alzheimer's disease and peripheral hard drusen formation [57].

8. Limitations of wide-field imaging systems

The eyeball is a three-dimensional structure. Since a two-dimensional image is obtained with a wide-field system, there are peripheral aberrations in the image. Because of the ellipsoid mirror used, lesions in the retinal periphery appear larger, with a slight distortion [58]. As this distortion and enlargement are variable in different directions, capturing should be done at the same direction as possible [24]. The Optomap system displays an area of 200° in the horizontal plane, while the vertical plane displays an area of 170° [58]. Evaluation of the retinal periphery, especially in the lower quadrant due to eyelashes, is difficult [1, 59]. **Figure 19** shows an image artifact caused by eyelashes.

Limitations of the Optos include laser artifacts, abnormal colors, and lack of stereopsis [9]. Also, resolution of the macula area is lower than that of standard fundus cameras [1]. Wide-angle retinal imaging with the use of a contact lens, such as the Staurenghi lens, expanded the view to 150° but is technically more challenging and requires high patient cooperation [12]. HRA is an alternative to Optos system in peripheral retinal imaging and each has its own advantages and disadvantages. A recent study has demonstrated that UWFA with the Optos system is able to capture a significantly wider total retinal area when compared to the Heidelberg noncontact system particularly in the nasal and temporal quadrants [60]. Although it was not found statistically significant, Heidelberg system was able to obtain a wider area in the superior and inferior quadrants. In contrast, Optos showed more peripheral distortion and greater variability in image quality, largely due to eyelash artifacts [60].

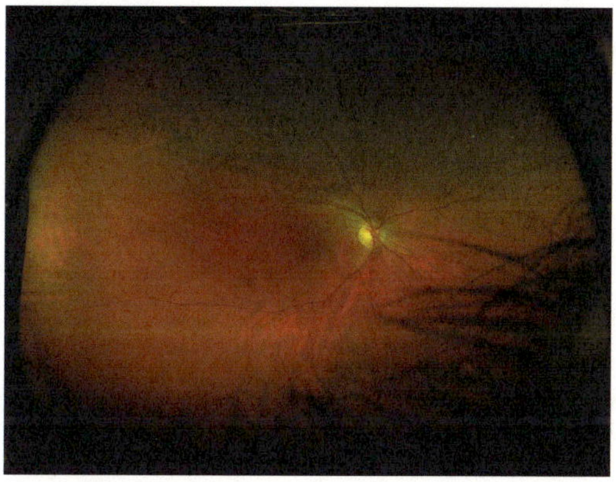

Figure 19.
Limited view in the lower quadrant due to eyelash artifacts.

9. Future directions

The future goal in retinal imaging is to capture a high-resolution image of the whole retina with the finest details. Devices that allow ultra-wide-field retinal imaging may be miniaturized, thus enhancing portability. These systems may also be integrated with smartphones, therefore facilitating telemedicine applications.

A novel smartphone-based wide-field retinal camera capable of capturing high-quality fundus images was previously described [61]. Nonphysician operators may also be trained to acquire retinal images for remote evaluation [62].

Different diagnostic tools embedded in one device will offer more cost- and time-efficient systems. A multimodal device combining conventional wide-field fundus photography, OCT, FA, FAF, ICGA, adaptive optics, and OCT angiography would be a step forward in retinal diagnostic testing. Incorporating a treatment utility such as laser photocoagulation into a multimodal diagnostic tool would be revolutionary in retina clinical practice.

10. Conclusion

The use of wide-field imaging systems for clinical applications and researches is increasing. In the future, the role of these imaging systems in the diagnosis, follow-up, and treatment of retinal diseases will continue to be demonstrated in comparative studies.

Acknowledgements

The authors would like to thank Dr. Eray Atalay for his help in final proof reading of the manuscript.

Conflict of interest

The authors declare that they do not have any financial conflict of interest related to the study.

Notes/thanks/other declarations

All images used in the section are from our archives of Optos and Retcam device.

Author details

Mustafa Değer Bilgeç[1], Nazmiye Erol[1] and Seyhan Topbaş[2]*

1 Ophthalmology Department, Eskisehir Osmangazi University Medical School, Eskisehir, Turkey

2 Private Umit Hospital Ophthalmology Department, Eskisehir, Turkey

*Address all correspondence to: stopbas@ogu.edu.tr

References

[1] Witmer MT, Kiss S. Wide-field imaging of the retina. Survey of Ophthalmology. 2013;**58**(2):143-154. DOI: 10.1016/j.survophthal.2012.07.003

[2] Sim DA, Keane PA, Rajendram R, Karampelas M, Selvam S, Powner MB, et al. Patterns of peripheral retinal and central macula ischemia in diabetic retinopathy as evaluated by ultra-widefield fluorescein angiography. American Journal of Ophthalmology. 2014;**158**(1):e141, 144-153. DOI: 10.1016/j.ajo.2014.03.009

[3] Diabetic Retinopathy Study. Report Number 6. Design, methods, and baseline results. Report Number 7. A modification of the Airlie House classification of diabetic retinopathy. Prepared by the Diabetic Retinopathy. Investigative Ophthalmology & Visual Science. 1981;**21**(1 Pt 2):1-226

[4] Manivannan A, Plskova J, Farrow A, McKay S, Sharp PF, Forrester JV. Ultra-wide-field fluorescein angiography of the ocular fundus. American Journal of Ophthalmology. 2005;**140**(3):525-527. DOI: 10.1016/j.ajo.2005.02.055

[5] Friberg TR, Gupta A, Yu J, Huang L, Suner I, Puliafito CA, et al. Ultrawide angle fluorescein angiographic imaging: A comparison to conventional digital acquisition systems. Ophthalmic Surgery, Lasers & Imaging. 2008;**39**(4):304-311

[6] Patel M, Kiss S. Ultra-wide-field fluorescein angiography in retinal disease. Current Opinion in Ophthalmology. 2014;**25**(3):213-220. DOI: 10.1097/ICU.0000000000000042

[7] Nagiel A, Lalane RA, Sadda SR, Schwartz SD. Ultra-widefield fundus imaging: A review of clinical applications and future trends. Retina. 2016;**36**(4):660-678. DOI: 10.1097/IAE.0000000000000937

[8] Mark HH. On the evolution of binocular ophthalmoscopy. Archives of Ophthalmology. 2007;**125**(6):830-833. DOI: 10.1001/archopht.125.6.830

[9] Leung EH, Rosen R. Fundus imaging in wide-field: A brief historical journey. In: Kozak I, Arévalo JF, editors. Atlas of Wide-Field Retinal Angiography and Imaging. 1st ed. Switzerland: Springer International Publishing; 2016. pp. 1-25. DOI: 10.1007/978-3-319-17864-6

[10] Pomerantzeff O. Wide-angle noncontact and small-angle contact cameras. Investigative Ophthalmology & Visual Science. 1980;**19**(8):973-979

[11] Shields CL, Materin M, Shields JA. Panoramic imaging of the ocular fundus. Archives of Ophthalmology. 2003;**121**(11):1603-1607. DOI: 10.1001/archopht.121.11.1603

[12] Staurenghi G, Viola F, Mainster MA, Graham RD, Harrington PG. Scanning laser ophthalmoscopy and angiography with a wide-field contact lens system. Archives of Ophthalmology. 2005;**123**(2):244-252. DOI: 10.1001/archopht.123.2.244

[13] Pomerantzeff O. Equator-plus camera. Investigative Ophthalmology. 1975;**14**(5):401-406

[14] Reeves GM, Kumar N, Beare NA, Pearce IA. Use of Staurenghi lens angiography in the management of posterior uveitis. Acta Ophthalmologica. 2013;**91**(1):48-51. DOI: 10.1111/j.1755-3768.2011.02200.x

[15] Dhaliwal C, Wright E, Graham C, McIntosh N, Fleck BW. Wide-field digital retinal imaging versus binocular indirect ophthalmoscopy for retinopathy of prematurity screening: A two-observer prospective, randomised comparison. The British Journal of

Ophthalmology. 2009;**93**(3):355-359. DOI: 10.1136/bjo.2008.148908

[16] Klufas MA, Yannuzzi NA, Pang CE, Srinivas S, Sadda SR, Freund KB, et al. Feasibility and clinical utility of ultra-widefield indocyanine green angiography. Retina. 2015;**35**(3):508-520. DOI: 10.1097/IAE.0000000000000318

[17] Yannuzzi LA, Ober MD, Slakter JS, Spaide RF, Fisher YL, Flower RW, et al. Ophthalmic fundus imaging: Today and beyond. American Journal of Ophthalmology. 2004;**137**(3):511-524. DOI: 10.1016/j.ajo.2003.12.035

[18] Erol N. Wide angle imaging: Technique, indications and assessment (analysis). Turkiye Klinikleri Journal of Ophthalmology. 2015;**8**(2):30-37

[19] Delori FC, Dorey CK, Staurenghi G, Arend O, Goger DG, Weiter JJ. In vivo fluorescence of the ocular fundus exhibits retinal pigment epithelium lipofuscin characteristics. Investigative Ophthalmology & Visual Science. 1995;**36**(3):718-729

[20] Heussen FM, Tan CS, Sadda SR. Prevalence of peripheral abnormalities on ultra-widefield greenlight (532 nm) autofluorescence imaging at a tertiary care center. Investigative Ophthalmology & Visual Science. 2012;**53**(10):6526-6531. DOI: 10.1167/iovs.12-9909

[21] Heussen FM, Puliafito CA, Sadda SR. Wide-field autofluorescence. In: Kozak I, Arévalo JF, editors. Atlas of Wide-Field Retinal Angiography and Imaging. 1st ed. Switzerland: Springer International Publishing; 2016. pp. 49-57. DOI: 10.1007/978-3-319-17864-6

[22] Pang CE, Shah VP, Sarraf D, Freund KB. Ultra-widefield imaging with autofluorescence and indocyanine green angiography in central serous chorioretinopathy. American Journal of Ophthalmology. 2014;**158**(2):362-371. e362. DOI: 10.1016/j.ajo.2014.04.021

[23] Lu J, Mai G, Luo Y, Li M, Cao D, Wang X, et al. Appearance of far peripheral retina in normal eyes by ultra-widefield fluorescein angiography. American Journal of Ophthalmology. 2017;**173**:84-90. DOI: 10.1016/j.ajo.2016.09.024

[24] Singer M, Sagong M, van Hemert J, Kuehlewein L, Bell D, Sadda SR. Ultra-widefield imaging of the peripheral retinal vasculature in normal subjects. Ophthalmology. 2016;**123**(5):1053-1059. DOI: 10.1016/j.ophtha.2016.01.022

[25] Shimizu K, Kobayashi Y, Muraoka K. Midperipheral fundus involvement in diabetic retinopathy. Ophthalmology. 1981;**88**(7):601-612

[26] Wessel MM, Aaker GD, Parlitsis G, Cho M, D'Amico DJ, Kiss S. Ultra-wide-field angiography improves the detection and classification of diabetic retinopathy. Retina. 2012;**32**(4):785-791. DOI: 10.1097/IAE.0b013e3182278b64

[27] Patel RD, Messner LV, Teitelbaum B, Michel KA, Hariprasad SM. Characterization of ischemic index using ultra-widefield fluorescein angiography in patients with focal and diffuse recalcitrant diabetic macular edema. American Journal of Ophthalmology. 2013;**155**(6):1038-1044 e 1032. DOI: 10.1016/j.ajo.2013.01.007

[28] Wessel MM, Nair N, Aaker GD, Ehrlich JR, D'Amico DJ, Kiss S. Peripheral retinal ischaemia, as evaluated by ultra-widefield fluorescein angiography, is associated with diabetic macular oedema. The British Journal of Ophthalmology. 2012;**96**(5):694-698. DOI: 10.1136/bjophthalmol-2011-300774

[29] Kernt M, Hadi I, Pinter F, Seidensticker F, Hirneiss C, Haritoglou C,

et al. Assessment of diabetic retinopathy using nonmydriatic ultra-widefield scanning laser ophthalmoscopy (Optomap) compared with ETDRS 7-field stereo photography. Diabetes Care. 2012;**35**(12):2459-2463. DOI: 10.2337/dc12-0346

[30] Silva PS, Cavallerano JD, Sun JK, Noble J, Aiello LM, Aiello LP. Nonmydriatic ultrawide field retinal imaging compared with dilated standard 7-field 35-mm photography and retinal specialist examination for evaluation of diabetic retinopathy. American Journal of Ophthalmology. 2012;**154**(3):549-559. e542. DOI: 10.1016/j.ajo.2012.03.019

[31] Rasmussen ML, Broe R, Frydkjaer-Olsen U, Olsen BS, Mortensen HB, Peto T, et al. Comparison between early treatment diabetic retinopathy study 7-field retinal photos and non-mydriatic, mydriatic and mydriatic steered widefield scanning laser ophthalmoscopy for assessment of diabetic retinopathy. Journal of Diabetes and its Complications. 2015;**29**(1):99-104. DOI: 10.1016/j.jdiacomp.2014.08.009

[32] Silva PS, Cavallerano JD, Sun JK, Soliman AZ, Aiello LM, Aiello LP. Peripheral lesions identified by mydriatic ultrawide field imaging: Distribution and potential impact on diabetic retinopathy severity. Ophthalmology. 2013;**120**(12):2587-2595. DOI: 10.1016/j.ophtha.2013.05.004

[33] Rogers S, McIntosh RL, Cheung N, Lim L, Wang JJ, Mitchell P, et al. The prevalence of retinal vein occlusion: Pooled data from population studies from the United States, Europe, Asia, and Australia. Ophthalmology. 2010;**117**(2):313-319, e311. DOI: 10.1016/j.ophtha.2009.07.017

[34] Tsui I, Bajwa A, Franco-Cardenas V, Pan CK, Kim HY, Schwartz SD. Peripheral fluorescein angiographic findings in fellow eyes of patients with branch retinal vein occlusion. International Journal of Inflammation. 2013;**2013**. DOI: 10.1155/2013/464127

[35] Prasad PS, Oliver SC, Coffee RE, Hubschman JP, Schwartz SD. Ultra wide-field angiographic characteristics of branch retinal and hemicentral retinal vein occlusion. Ophthalmology. 2010;**117**(4):780-784. DOI: 10.1016/j.ophtha.2009.09.019

[36] Noma H, Minamoto A, Funatsu H, Tsukamoto H, Nakano K, Yamashita H, et al. Intravitreal levels of vascular endothelial growth factor and interleukin-6 are correlated with macular edema in branch retinal vein occlusion. Graefe's Archive for Clinical and Experimental Ophthalmology. 2006;**244**(3):309-315. DOI: 10.1007/s00417-004-1087-4

[37] Tsui I, Prasad PS. Wide-field retinal imaging of central retinal vein occlusions. In: Kozak I, Arévalo JF, editors. Atlas of Wide-Field Retinal Angiography and Imaging. 1st ed. Switzerland: Springer International Publishing; 2016. pp. 83-91. DOI: 10.1007/978-3-319-17864-6

[38] Spaide RF. Peripheral areas of nonperfusion in treated central retinal vein occlusion as imaged by wide-field fluorescein angiography. Retina. 2011;**31**(5):829-837. DOI: 10.1097/IAE.0b013e31820c841e

[39] Tsui I, Kaines A, Havunjian MA, Hubschman S, Heilweil G, Prasad PS, et al. Ischemic index and neovascularization in central retinal vein occlusion. Retina. 2011;**31**(1):105-110. DOI: 10.1097/IAE.0b013e3181e36c6d

[40] Jain A, Shah SP, Tsui I, McCannel TA. The value of Optos Panoramic 200MA imaging for the monitoring of large suspicious choroidal lesions. Seminars in Ophthalmology.

2009;**24**(1):43-44. DOI: 10.1080/08820530802520384

[41] Kernt M, Schaller UC, Stumpf C, Ulbig MW, Kampik A, Neubauer AS. Choroidal pigmented lesions imaged by ultra-wide-field scanning laser ophthalmoscopy with two laser wavelengths (Optomap). Clinical Ophthalmology. 2010;**4**:829-836

[42] Coffee RE, Jain A, McCannel TA. Ultra wide-field imaging of choroidal metastasis secondary to primary breast cancer. Seminars in Ophthalmology. 2009;**24**(1):34-36. DOI: 10.1080/08820530802520194

[43] Kornberg DL, Klufas MA, Yannuzzi NA, Orlin A, D'Amico DJ, Kiss S. Clinical utility of ultra-widefield imaging with the optos optomap compared with indirect ophthalmoscopy in the setting of non-traumatic rhegmatogenous retinal detachment. Seminars in Ophthalmology. 2016;**31**(5):505-512. DOI: 10.3109/08820538.2014.981551

[44] Reznicek L, Wasfy T, Stumpf C, Kampik A, Ulbig M, Neubauer AS, et al. Peripheral fundus autofluorescence is increased in age-related macular degeneration. Investigative Ophthalmology & Visual Science. 2012;**53**(4):2193-2198. DOI: 10.1167/iovs.11-8483

[45] Tan CS, Heussen F, Sadda SR. Peripheral autofluorescence and clinical findings in neovascular and non-neovascular age-related macular degeneration. Ophthalmology. 2013;**120**(6):1271-1277. DOI: 10.1016/j.ophtha.2012.12.002

[46] Patel CK, Fung TH, Muqit MM, Mordant DJ, Brett J, Smith L, et al. Non-contact ultra-widefield imaging of retinopathy of prematurity using the Optos dual wavelength scanning laser ophthalmoscope. Eye (London, England). 2013;**27**(5):589-596. DOI: 10.1038/eye.2013.45

[47] Scott KE, Kim DY, Wang L, Kane SA, Coki O, Starren J, et al. Telemedical diagnosis of retinopathy of prematurity intraphysician agreement between ophthalmoscopic examination and image-based interpretation. Ophthalmology. 2008;**115**(7):1222-1228e 1223. DOI: 10.1016/j.ophtha.2007.09.006

[48] Kang KB, Orlin A, Lee TC, Chiang MF, Chan RV. The use of digital imaging in the identification of skip areas after laser treatment for retinopathy of prematurity and its implications for education and patient care. Retina. 2013;**33**(10):2162-2169. DOI: 10.1097/IAE.0b013e31828e6969

[49] Tsui I, Franco-Cardenas V, Hubschman JP, Schwartz SD. Pediatric retinal conditions imaged by ultra wide field fluorescein angiography. Ophthalmic Surgery, Lasers and Imaging Retina. 2013;**44**(1):59-67. DOI: 10.3928/23258160-20121221-14

[50] Kang KB, Wessel MM, Tong J, D'Amico DJ, Chan RV. Ultra-widefield imaging for the management of pediatric retinal diseases. Journal of Pediatric Ophthalmology and Strabismus. 2013;**50**(5):282-288. DOI: 10.3928/01913913-20130528-04

[51] Kashani AH, Brown KT, Chang E, Drenser KA, Capone A, Trese MT. Diversity of retinal vascular anomalies in patients with familial exudative vitreoretinopathy. Ophthalmology. 2014;**121**(11):2220-2227. DOI: 10.1016/j.ophtha.2014.05.029

[52] Campbell JP, Leder HA, Sepah YJ, Gan T, Dunn JP, Hatef E, et al. Wide-field retinal imaging in the management of noninfectious posterior uveitis. American Journal of Ophthalmology. 2012;**154**(5):908-911, e902. DOI: 10.1016/j.ajo.2012.05.019

[53] Tsui I, Kaines A, Schwartz S. Patterns of periphlebitis in intermediate uveitis using ultra wide field fluorescein angiography. Seminars in Ophthalmology. 2009;**24**(1):29-33. DOI: 10.1080/08820530802520186

[54] Kaines A, Tsui I, Sarraf D, Schwartz S. The use of ultra wide field fluorescein angiography in evaluation and management of uveitis. Seminars in Ophthalmology. 2009;**24**(1):19-24. DOI: 10.1080/08820530802520095

[55] Mesquida M, Llorenc V, Fontenla JR, Navarro MJ, Adan A. Use of ultra-wide-field retinal imaging in the management of active Behcet retinal vasculitis. Retina. 2014;**34**(10):2121-2127. DOI: 10.1097/IAE.0000000000000197

[56] Kaneko Y, Moriyama M, Hirahara S, Ogura Y, Ohno-Matsui K. Areas of nonperfusion in peripheral retina of eyes with pathologic myopia detected by ultra-widefield fluorescein angiography. Investigative Ophthalmology & Visual Science. 2014;**55**(3):1432-1439. DOI: 10.1167/iovs.13-13706

[57] Csincsik L, Mac Gillivray TJ, Flynn E, Pellegrini E, Papanastasiou G, Barzegar-Befroei N, et al. Peripheral retinal imaging biomarkers for Alzheimer's disease: A pilot study. Ophthalmic Research. 2018;**59**(4): 182-192. DOI: 10.1159/000487053

[58] Oishi A, Hidaka J, Yoshimura N. Quantification of the image obtained with a wide-field scanning ophthalmoscope. Investigative Ophthalmology & Visual Science. 2014;**55**(4):2424-2431. DOI: 10.1167/iovs.13-13738

[59] Mackenzie PJ, Russell M, Ma PE, Isbister CM, Maberley DA. Sensitivity and specificity of the optos optomap for detecting peripheral retinal lesions. Retina. 2007;**27**(8):1119-1124. DOI: 10.1097/IAE.0b013e3180592b5c

[60] Witmer MT, Parlitsis G, Patel S, Kiss S. Comparison of ultra-widefield fluorescein angiography with the Heidelberg Spectralis((R)) noncontact ultra-widefield module versus the Optos((R)) Optomap((R)). Clinical Ophthalmology. 2013;7:389-394. DOI: 10.2147/OPTH.S41731

[61] Maamari RN, Keenan JD, Fletcher DA, Margolis TP. A mobile phone-based retinal camera for portable wide field imaging. The British Journal of Ophthalmology. 2014;**98**(4):438-441. DOI: 10.1136/bjophthalmol-2013-303797

[62] Fijalkowski N, Zheng LL, Henderson MT, Wang SK, Wallenstein MB, Leng T, et al. Stanford University Network for Diagnosis of Retinopathy of Prematurity (SUNDROP): Five years of screening with telemedicine. Ophthalmic Surgery, Lasers and Imaging Retina. 2014;**45**(2):106-113. DOI: 10.3928/23258160-20140122-01

Chapter 5

A Brief Overview of Ophthalmic Ultrasound Imaging

David B. Rosen, Mandi D. Conway, Charles P. Ingram, Robin D. Ross, Leonardo G. Montilla and Gholam A. Peyman

Abstract

Ultrasound is one of the oldest imaging modalities. Sound waves are emitted into the body, and the returning echoes can be interpreted. It has become widely used because it can easily be done at bedside with a relatively small apparatus and does not expose the patient to any ionizing radiation. While this technique has seen widespread acceptance in other fields such as cardiology or obstetrics and gynecology, the general use in ophthalmology has been somewhat limited. However, recent advancements in ultrasonic arrays can be a powerful tool in the evaluation of ophthalmic pathology. Such systems can quickly generate very high detail images and 3D reconstructions without the need for extensive manual scanning. The application of this technology includes evaluation of traumatic eye injuries; assessing presence and location of an intraocular foreign body; evaluation of intraocular tumors, including small tumors that have not yet caused visual distortion; evaluation of retinal detachment; and evaluation of vascular disease. The goal of this article is to briefly review the history and development of ultrasound and to provide an overview of the most current systems and applications of ultrasound use in ophthalmologic clinical evaluation.

Keywords: ultrasound, 3D reconstruction, ultrasonic biomicroscopy, Doppler ultrasonography, ultrasonic array

1. Introduction

One of the most common and well recognized technologies in modern medicine is ultrasonography. Its use has been used in many medical fields, and new methods and devices using ultrasound are frequently emerging. While there have been many recent advancements, ultrasound has a rich history dating back centuries.

Some consider the earliest investigation into ultrasound beginning with the ancient Greeks [1]. Pythagoras invented the sonometer to study music; Boethius compared the waves generated by dropping a pebble into water to sound waves.

In 1880, French scientists and brothers, Pierre and Jacques Curie, discovered piezoelectricity [2]. When certain materials (such as some crystals) are exposed to an electric field they undergo mechanical changes. The reverse is also true: when piezoelectric materials have mechanical force exerted on them they generate an electric charge. Thus, these crystals can both transmit and receive sound. Such piezoelectric devices are the basis of ultrasound transducers [3]. When voltage is applied to the transducer sound waves are emitted; when the reflected waves are picked up by the transducer, they generate voltage. This electrical signal can then be processed to produce an "image" based on the reflected sound waves.

While the Curie brothers discovered the piezoelectric effect in the 1880s, it wasn't utilized for ultrasonography until a few decades later. One of their students, Paul Langevin, was commissioned by the French government to develop technology to detect enemy submarines [2]. His studies became the base for what was to later become known as sound navigation ranging (SONAR), which was developed extensively in World War II [4, 5].

Later, ultrasound started to see use in medicine. Karl Dussik used it to study brain tissue; George Ludwig used ultrasound to help detect gallstones [2]. In 1951, John Wild and John Reid built the first B-mode scanner [6]. B-mode (brightness-mode) scanners are what is most often thought of when one refers to ultrasound. B-mode produces a two-dimensional reconstructed image of internal body structures based on reflected sound waves. The first commercially available handheld B-mode scanner was produced in 1963 [6]. Around the same time, many researchers started looking into Doppler applications with ultrasound to detect blood flow as well.

The 1960s and 1970s proved to be a time of rapid development for the use of ultrasound in medicine [2, 6]. Its application in cardiology and obstetrics and gynecology became more widespread. The field of medical sonography continued to grow, and various societies and institutions dedicated to medical sonography began to emerge.

2. Ultrasound use in ophthalmology

In the 1950s, ultrasound was first used in ophthalmology and optometry [7, 8]. These early explorations aimed at using measurements of the depth and velocity of sound waves in the eye to try to distinguish various conditions. This type of ultrasonography is known as A-scanning (amplitude scanning). Further advances in the 1960s used A-mode scanning to better measure the length of the eye, distances within the eye [9], and visual axis of the eye [10]. The axial A-scanning was also used to help determine intraocular lens power [11]. Diagnostic A-scan works by emitting a sonic pulse and measuring the time and amplitude of the echo. This information can then be interpreted to give information on the number of interfaces the wave has passed through. For example, the waveform produced from passing through normal structures of the eye versus a hemangioma versus a more solid lesion will all look different [7]. While A-scanning can give important data on some basic characteristics of the eye, such as lens power and length of the eye, it does not produce a visual re-creation of internal ocular structures. Because of this, its use is somewhat limited and must be combined with B-scan (**Figures 1** and **2**).

Another valuable application of ultrasound is the use of Doppler flow ultrasonography. Doppler was a physicist and astronomer in the mid 1800s who demonstrated that blue stars appeared that color because they were moving toward the observer while red stars appeared red because they were moving away from the observer [12]. This became known as the Doppler effect, and held true not only for electromagnetic waves but also acoustic waves; thus, the Doppler effect can be applied to ultrasound to help measure the magnitude and direction of flow.

Doppler found early application in cardiology, where the evaluation of flow was obvious [13, 14]. Doppler ultrasound soon found other applications, though. It proved useful in monitoring and measuring peripheral vasculature [15–18]. This proved useful for applications such as detecting tumor neovascularization [19, 20] and evaluation for ectopic pregnancy [21].

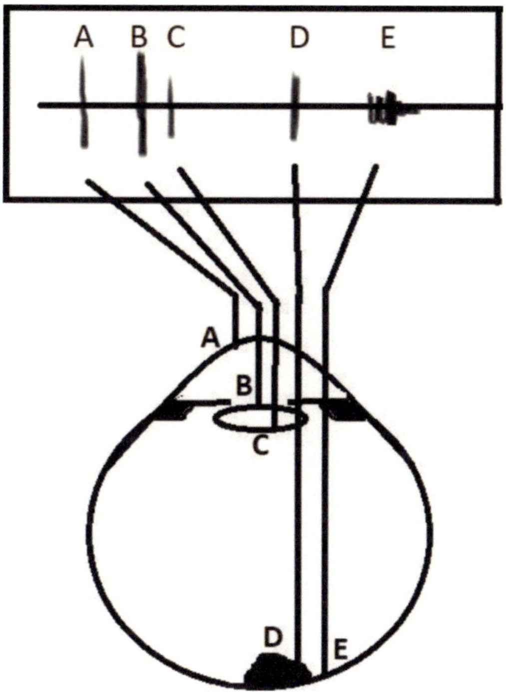

Figure 1.
A diagram illustrating the various sources of reflected waves within the eye and how they would appear on the view screen.

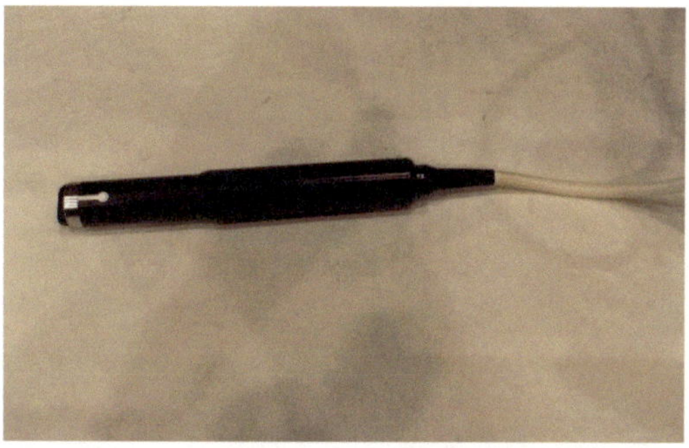

Figure 2.
Example of an ultrasound probe designed specifically for ophthalmic use.

Doppler ultrasonography was also shown to be useful in estimating the degree of stenosis in vasculature, which proved especially useful in evaluating carotid artery disease [22]. This is of special interest because the ophthalmic artery is the first branch of the internal carotid artery, and disease affecting the internal carotid has the propensity to affect ocular vasculature either indirectly secondary to decreased flow or directly through embolism of atherosclerotic plaque [23]. Doppler was also shown to be helpful in diagnosis and evaluation of open angle glaucoma [24]. Doppler has also been used in ophthalmology to evaluate the ocular fundus [25] and flow through the retinal artery [26].

While A-mode scanning and Doppler flow ultrasound had their specific uses, B-mode scanning was explored more broadly. Devices became more accessible with handheld transducers and options to attach to a TV screen for viewing [27, 28]. In addition, differently shaped probes were developed to aid in imaging for different surface areas or structures [29]. B-mode proved an invaluable tool for evaluating intraocular foreign bodies, masses, hemorrhage, retinal detachment, and congenital abnormalities. It was first pioneered in ophthalmology Baum and Greenwood [30], and the first ocular specific probe was produced by Bronson [27].

One of the first ways B-mode ultrasonography was used in ophthalmology was for evaluation of an opaque eye [30]. For example, if there is a potential foreign body in the eye and there is clouding of the cornea or lens, the object may not be able to be observed directly. Furthermore, if it is radio-opaque, it will not be visible via X-ray. This makes ultrasound an excellent modality for evaluation in such instances. Another advantage is that ultrasonographic evaluation of the eye can be done bedside with the need for minimal equipment, making it ideal for traumatic evaluation [31–33].

B-mode was also used early on for evaluation of intraocular tumors [34–36]. Similar to the above example of foreign object location, if there is a soft tissue lesion that is in a position not easily visible by direct ophthalmoscopy or if there is clouding of anterior structures, such that a direct view is not possible, B-mode ultrasonography can aide in evaluation of intraocular soft tissue masses (**Figure 3**). This has been especially explored in the setting of diagnosing choroidal melanoma [37]. B-mode scanning can help ascertain the position, size, and height of ocular melanoma.

While early scans for evaluation of intraocular masses were focused on identifying presence and location, later research focused on better quantifying such tumors [38, 39]. By taking serial cross-sectional scans over the shape of the tumor, the shape and volume of the tumor could be estimated [40, 41]. This helped to improve evaluation and characterization of intraocular masses and guided radioactive plaque placement.

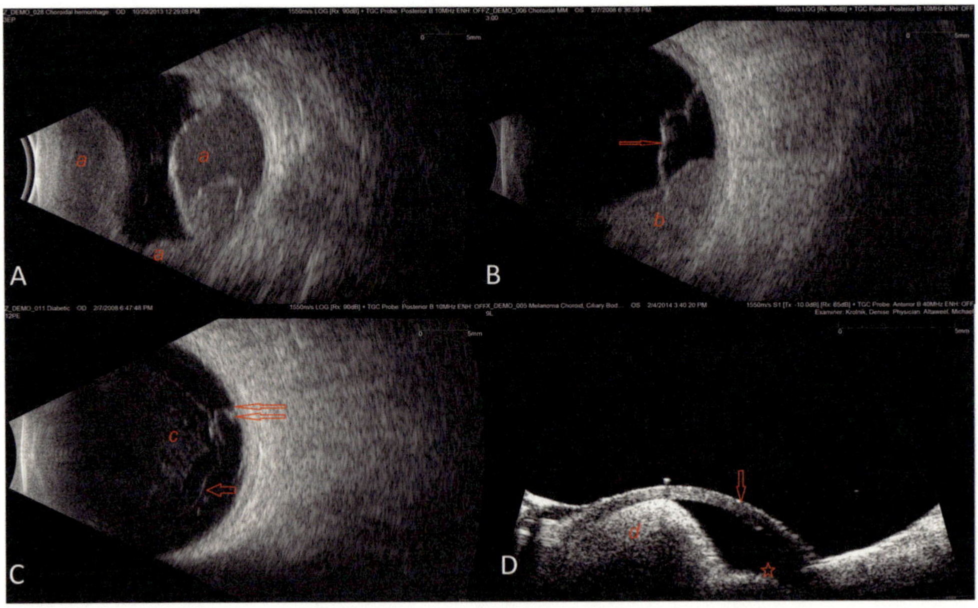

Figure 3.
Examples of images from B-scan ultrasound. (A) An image of choroidal hemorrhage. Areas of hemorrhage indicated by (a). (B) Choroidal melanoma (b) with associated superior retinal detachment (arrow). (C) A diabetic patient with vitreous retinal traction. Area of vitreous hemorrhage shown by (c); single arrow indicates posterior hyaloid membrane; double arrow shows point of fibrovascular adhesion. (D) Ciliary melanoma (d) invading into the anterior chamber; arrow indicates cornea while star shows the location of the iris. Images used courtesy of Ellex.

Despite the many applications of ultrasonography for ocular evaluation, there are some limitations. The depth of penetration of ultrasonic waves is inversely proportional to the frequency used [42]; a transducer using a 10 MHz frequency can penetrate 50 mm, where as a system using 60 MHz frequency will only penetrate 5 mm. Furthermore, the image resolution is limited by the frequency used, with higher frequency systems achieving higher resolution images. Ultrasonic imaging using high frequencies has been termed "ultrasonic microscopy" or "ultrasonic backscatter microscopy" (UBM) [43, 44]. Such systems use very high frequency waves (60-100 MHz) to achieve high resolution images at depths in the 4 mm range. This technique is ideal for high resolution imaging the anterior chamber, ciliary body and its structures, as well as parts of the peripheral retina [45]. Because images can get distorted at the close interface between the transducer and the object being imaged, eye-cup devices are used to create an offset distance between the transducer and the surface of what is being imaged (**Figure 4**) [42].

The use of high frequency ultrasonic biomicroscopy has been applied in several ways. One study used UBM for tracking corneal changes related to the laser-assisted in-situ keratomileusis (LASIK) procedure [46]. 50 MHz scanning was used to map the cornea before and after LASIK. They showed that this technique was an accurate and feasible way to track changes in corneal shape and thickness following LASIK. Another application of ultrasonic biomicroscopy was the characterization of the lens [47]. By being able to better characterize the natural lens, more accurate synthetic lenses can be produced (**Figure 5**). A similar approach was used to better categorize the ciliary body [48]. In contrast to anterior structures such as the cornea and lens can be easily evaluated via direct visualization with methods such as slit lamp examination, the ciliary body is obscured from direct visual view. Because of this, UBM is an ideal modality for evaluation of ciliary body pathology, small tumors in particular [49–51]. UBM has also been useful in identifying structural morphologies contributing to glaucoma, such as iris plateau syndrome [52]. These examples illustrate how high frequency, high resolution ultrasonic biomicroscopy can practically be applied to ocular evaluation and how this imaging can change practice and drive innovation.

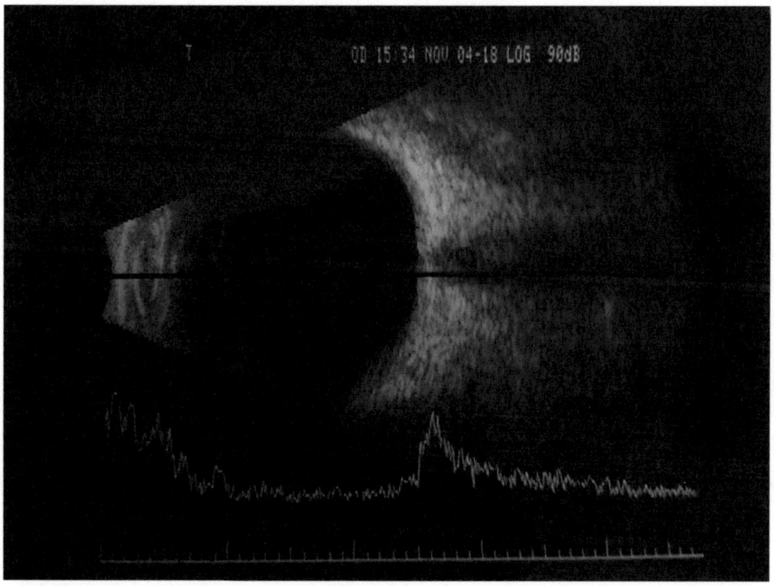

Figure 4.
The 2D image is an example of B-scan ultrasonography of a human eye. The lower section of the image shows a superimposed A-scan for comparison.

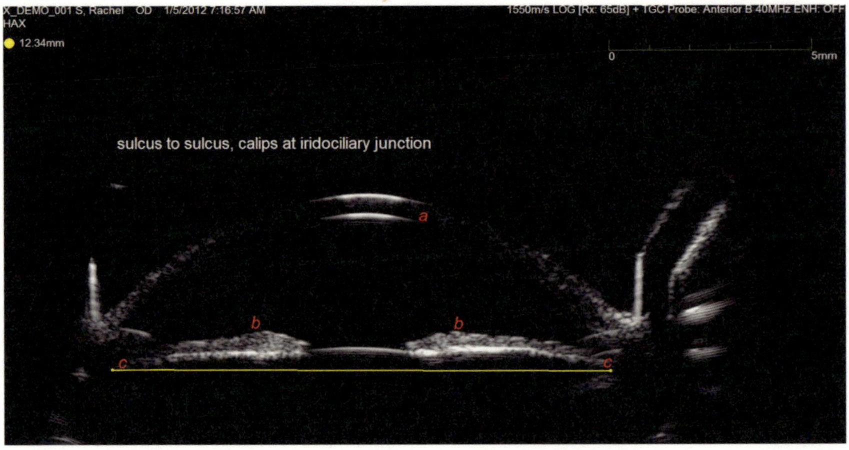

Figure 5.
Example of UBM for visualization of anterior structures. Cornea indicated by (a), iris by (b), and ciliary body by (c). This technique can be used for measurements for intraocular lens placement, or to assess ciliary body tumors which would not be directly visible. Image used courtesy of Ellex.

Despite advances in high resolution imaging and faster B-scanning, there were still limitations. One is that ultrasonic evaluation can be time consuming and the quality of the exam is dependent of how skillful the examiner is. Another limitation is that traditional B-mode scanning can only evaluate structures directly opposite to the probe and cannot provide information in the XY plane without 3D reconstruction. While 3D reconstruction was shown to be possible [40, 41] and could give information about the XY planes, such imaging required time consuming serial acquisition of small 2D image slices and subsequent reconstruction. This meant that while 3D reconstruction is possible, it is too cumbersome to be used frequently in the average clinical setting. Much research went into designing systems that were able to scan faster to produce more reliable 3D reconstructions of ocular models [53, 54]. This included using array systems that were able to image at both high frequencies and traditional frequencies to obtain a reconstruction with as much detail as possible at multiple depths [54]. As opposed to traditional A-mode and B-mode transducers which have a single piezoelectric element (and thereby a fixed depth of focus), arrays use a transducer with many elements (over 100) in each transducer head [55].

Despite the valuable information that can be gained from an array system that utilizes both traditional and high frequency waves, such systems have not been readily adopted [56, 57]. One potential reason for the underutilization of high frequency systems may be because of the equipment constraints. Because array transducers require over 100 piezoelectric parts aligned in close proximity within a relatively small transducer head, the production is technically challenging [55, 58]. Moreover, the frequency generated is inversely proportional to the size and spacing of the piezoelectric elements [58]: lower frequency systems can use larger more widely spaced piezoelectric crystals.

A combined low and high frequency array system called the Vevo 2100 (VisualSonics, Toronto, Ontario, Canada) has been tested for use in ophthalmologic evaluation and shows promise [55]. This system uses an array transducer with 256 elements in each transducer head. By utilizing an array system, most of the imaged field can be kept in focus, allowing high-resolution real-time imaging. This system has two linear array transducer probes: a 25 MHz probe and a 50 MHz probe (**Figure 6**). This system generates 3D reconstructions in seconds utilizing a mechanical motor for efficient scanning. A scan using the 50 MHz probe yields high definition data on the anterior eye structures, while a second scan using the 25 MHz probe will

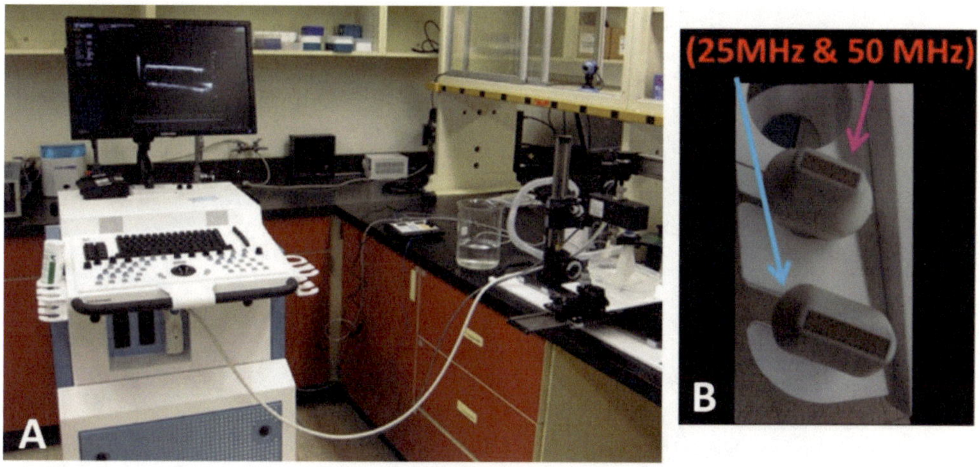

Figure 6.
(A) Picture of the Vevo 2100 system (VisualSonics, Toronto, Ontario, Canada). (B) Picture of the 25 MHz and 50 MHz probe utilized by this system. Used with permission from Gholam A. Peyman.

produce data on the posterior segment and orbit. Each scan with 3D reconstruction takes about 10 seconds. An initial evaluation would be a scan with the 50 MHz transducer to assess anterior structures followed by a scan using the 25 MHz probe to image the rest of the eye. By choosing an appropriate transducer and frequency, the whole eye can efficiently be scanned, and a 3D reconstruction generated either from a specific area or the whole eye in less than 1 minute. In addition to generation of 3D reconstructions (**Figures** 7 and **8**), this system can perform several other scanning functions, including B-mode, M-mode, PW Doppler, Color Doppler, Power Doppler, Tissue Doppler, Contrast Mode, and Photoacoustic Imaging.

One important application of this system is in emergency evaluation of traumatic eye injuries. Traditional hand-held B-mode evaluation is an excellent tool for detecting foreign bodies but is not without risk. Extreme caution must be used when scanning an injured eye, which must be considered as a potential open globe. It is critical to avoid placing pressure and extruding intraocular contents through a penetrating wound. This system can perform a mechanized scan through a closed eyelid with a coupling medium. There is decreased risk of causing further injury to the eye. This feature, combined with the high-resolution 3D reconstruction, will provide detailed information in seconds on the extent of ocular injury, presence and position of a foreign body (**Figure 9**).

This system is also useful for routine clinical outpatient evaluation. The 50 MHz transducer can provide a very high level of detail on eyelid, including Meibomian glands (**Figure 10**), and anterior ocular structures: cornea, iris, ciliary body, and lens. Because of the very high level of resolution, it could be a powerful tool for assessing Meibomian gland disease. By using this scan routinely, small tumors or lesions behind the iris or in the choroid may be detected early, before they caused visual distortion or metastases. Small retinal detachments at the peripheral retina can also be detected using this transducer. This may be very helpful in children with retinal detachment.

In summary, the 50 MHz transducer can provide fine detail of anterior structures, a subsequent scan using the 25 MHz transducer can provide information on the remainder of the eye. This is useful for assessment in the setting of trauma, additionally it can also provide valuable information on retinal detachment, size and location of intraocular masses, and information on the optic nerve head drusen or edema. Because this system can provide simultaneous B-mode scanning and Doppler flow imaging, both anatomic assessment and evaluation of vascular disease

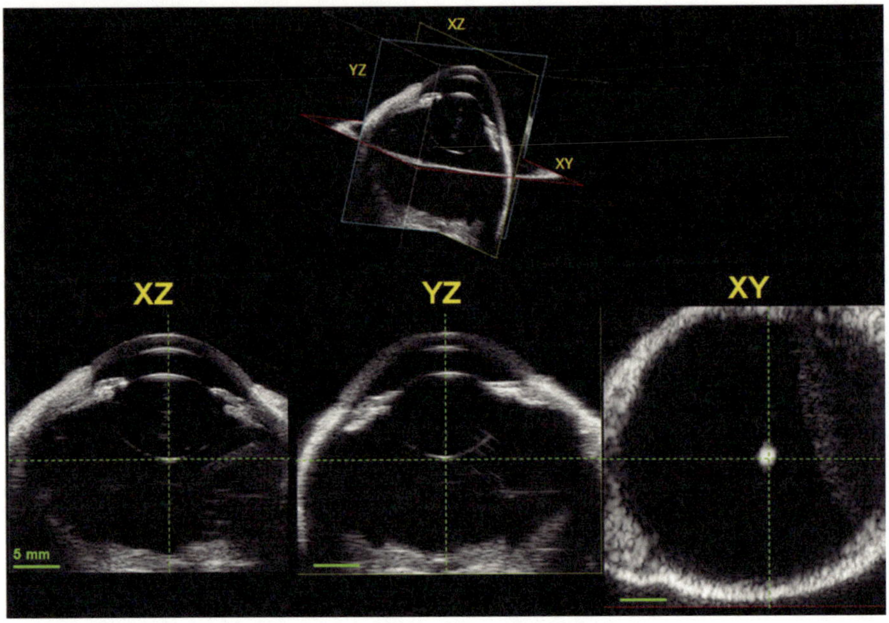

Figure 7.
The lower panels depict 2D slices of a pig eye in different planes obtained with the 25 MHz probe. The upper image is a 3D perspective. Used with permission from Gholam A. Peyman.

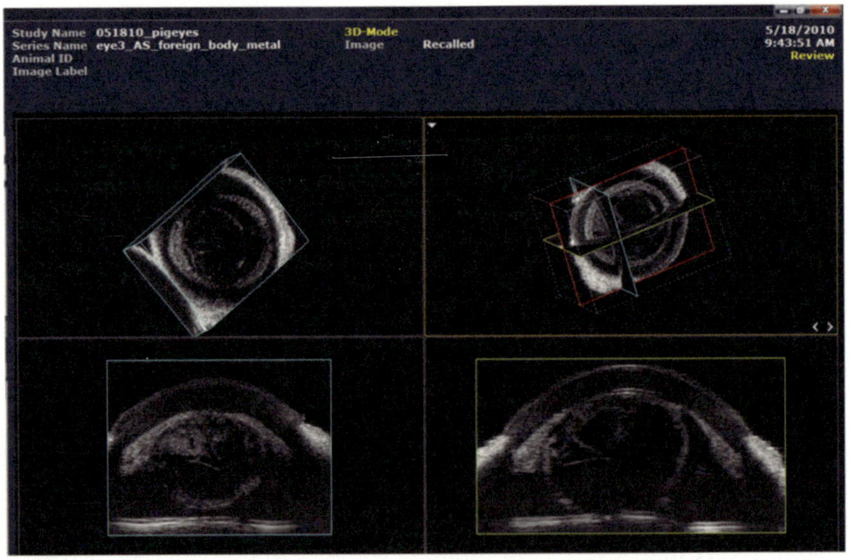

Figure 8.
Example of 3D reconstruction of a pig eye with anterior lens injury. Various planes are shown. Used with permission from Gholam A. Peyman.

of the optic nerve head can be performed. Doppler flow imaging can also be utilized to assess other vascular diseases, such as temporal arteritis (**Figure 11**).

Overall, the Vevo 2100 system (VisualSonics, Toronto, Ontario, Canada) potentially is a powerful tool for emergency and routine evaluation of ophthalmic pathology. By utilizing an array system in the transducer head, real-time images well focused throughout the scan may be obtained. The mechanical scanning function can produce 3D models in seconds with decreased risk of expulsion of

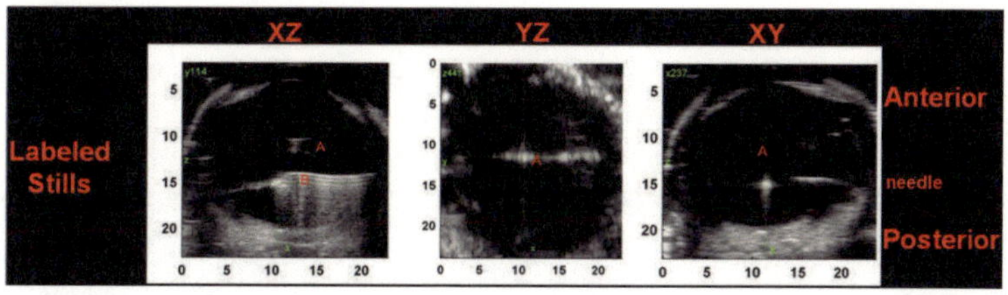

Figure 9.
This image shows the presence of a linear foreign body (A) and secondary acoustic shadowing (B). The images were generated using Matlab (Mathworks, Natick, MA) and a point-and-click technique in which an object is found in one plane, clicked on, and automatically images in the two other planes are generated. used with permission from Gholam A. Peyman.

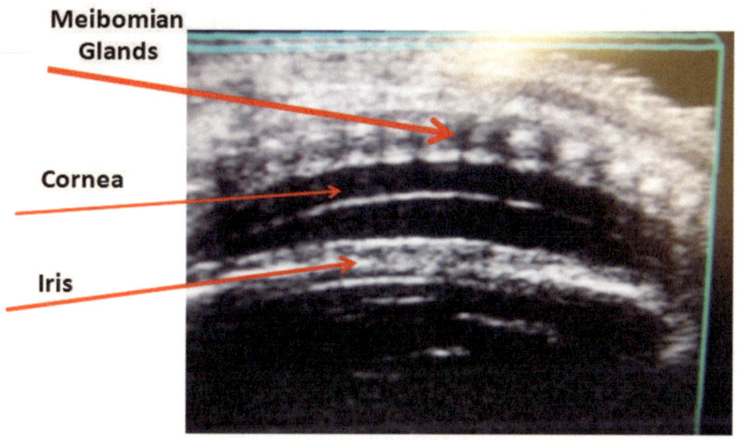

Figure 10.
Image obtained from a scan using the 50 MHz transducer. Structures visible, including the Meibomian glands, are labeled. used with permission from Gholam A. Peyman.

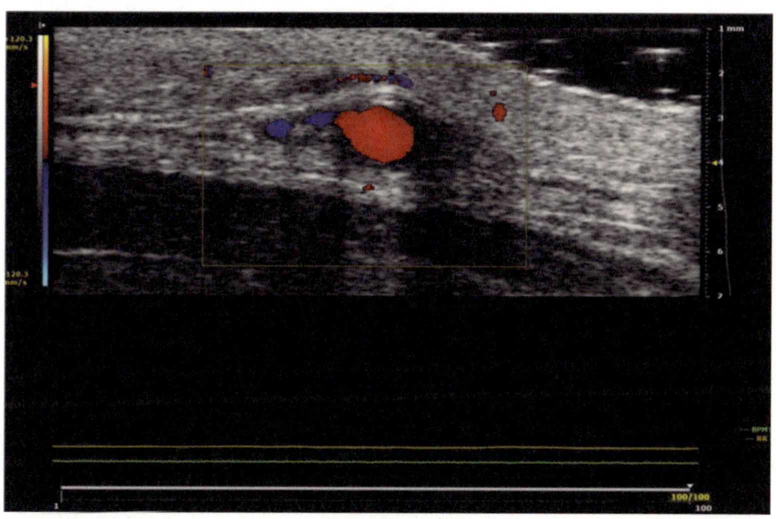

Figure 11.
Example of color Doppler image showing flow through temporal artery. Obtained using 50 MHz transducer. Used with permission from Gholam A. Peyman.

ocular contents following trauma. These 3D reconstructions provide information in planes traditional B-scanning methods cannot assess. The level of detail produced using this system can provide information on a wide array of ocular disease, from

Meibomian gland, evaluation of intraocular tumors or foreign bodies, vascular diseases affecting the optic nerve head, glaucomatous cupping, drusen and optic nerve edema as well as orbital tumors (**Figure 12** and **Table 1**).

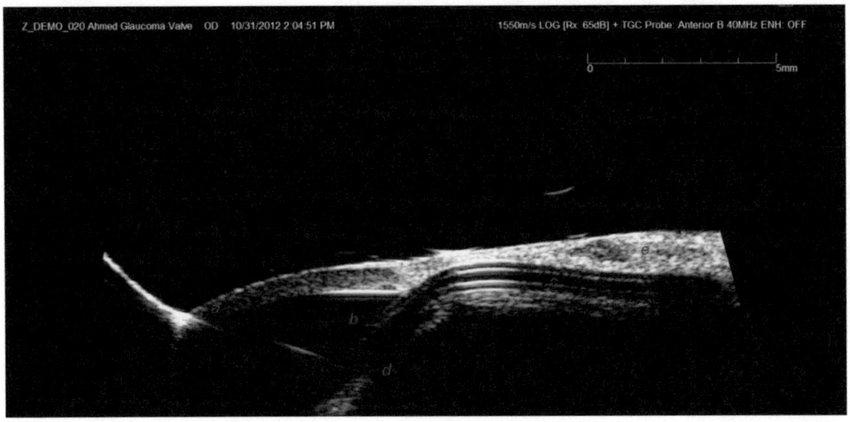

Figure 12.
Example of an ultrasound image showing the correct placement of an Ahmed valve for treatment of glaucoma. The cornea is visible (a) with the tip of the valve in the anterior chamber (b) with the iris labeled (d). The main tubing (c) lies within the sclera (e).

Clinical uses of ocular ultrasonography	
Use	**Clinical comment**
Intraocular foreign bodies (see **Figure 9**)	• Ideal for emergent evaluation of traumatic eye. • Can detect objects in periphery (not easily seen on direct visualization). • 3D reconstruction can yield detailed information on size and location.
Intraocular tumors (see **Figure 3B**)	• Useful in diagnosing intraocular soft tissue masses. • Can detect malignant melanoma.
Vascular disease	• Doppler can be used to assess flow through ocular vasculature. • Evaluate condition of retinal artery. • Evaluation of temporal arteritis.
Ciliary body pathology (see **Figure 5**)	• UBM provides fine level of detail. • Can be used to assess ciliary body disease. • Can detect ciliary body tumors that cannot be directly observed.
Structural changes in glaucoma (see **Figure 12**)	• Detect iris plateau syndrome. • Assess glaucoma drainage devices. • Measurement of anterior chamber depth. • Evaluate optic nerve cupping.
Evaluation of an opaque eye (see **Figure 3A**)	• Evaluation of pathology that could ordinarily be directly visible such as: ○ Retinal detachment ○ Vitreous hemorrhage ○ Presence and location of foreign bodies or tumors ○ Glaucomatous cupping ○ Optic nerve edema

Table 1.
Examples of clinical applications of ultrasonic evaluation in ophthalmology.

3. Conclusion

Ultrasound is an established diagnostic imaging modality. There are many systems which are relatively small with handheld probes. No ionizing radiation is used, but the image resolution can be limited compared to other visualization modalities. Advances have allowed high resolution imaging possible, especially of the anterior segment with the ability to create 3D reconstructions of ocular tissues and foreign bodies to aid in diagnosis and management of many disorders. Doppler flow can be an invaluable tool in the real time diagnosis of vasculopathies. However, 3D systems with rapid scan acquisition are not yet readily available.

Acknowledgements

The authors thank Global Retina Institute for providing funding and for Ellex, Inc for use of ultrasound images.

Conflict of interest

No author has a conflict of interest related to this work.

Abbreviations

SONAR	sound navigation imaging
UBM	ultrasonic backscatter microscopy
LASIK	laser-assisted in-situ keratomileusis

Author details

David B. Rosen[1], Mandi D. Conway[1,2*], Charles P. Ingram[3], Robin D. Ross[1,4], Leonardo G. Montilla[3] and Gholam A. Peyman[1,2,5]

1 Department of Ophthalmology, University of Arizona College of Medicine, USA

2 Department of Ophthalmology, Tulane University College of Medicine, USA

3 Department of Radiology, University of Arizona, Tucson, Arizona, USA

4 Department of Bioethics and Medical Humanism, University of Arizona College of Medicine, Phoenix, Arizona, USA

5 College of Optical Sciences, University of Arizona, USA

*Address all correspondence to: mconway1@yahoo.com

References

[1] Baker J. Ultrasound history. Radiology Today 2008;**9**:28. Available from: https://www.radiologytoday.net/archive/rt_120108p28.shtml [Accessed: October 27, 2018]

[2] Baker JP. The history of sonographers. Journal of Ultrasound in Medicine. 2005;**24**:1-14. DOI: 10.7863/jum.2005.24.1.1

[3] Moeller D-PF. Whitepaper-ultrasound PIEZO elements IN medical technology. Ultrasound Piezo Elements in Medical Technology Tool, Therapeutic Device and Sensor. Karlsruhe. n.d.

[4] Kimmelman B. Medical Diagnostic Ultrasound: A Retrosepctive on its 40th Anniversary. Bethesda: Eastman Kodak Co; American Institue of Ultrasound in Medicine; 1988

[5] Craig M. Introduction to Ultrasonography and Patient Care. Philadelphia: WB Saunders Co; 1993

[6] Hagen-Ansert SL. Society of diagnostic medical sonographers—A timeline of historical events in sonography and the development of the SDMS: In the beginning.... Journal of Diagnostic Medical Sonography. 2006;**22**:272-278. DOI: 10.1177/8756479306291456

[7] Mundt GH, Mundt GH, Hughes WF. Ultrasonics in ocular diagnosis.pdf. American Journal of Ophthalmology. 1956;**41**:488-498. DOI: 10.1016/0002-9394(56)91262-4

[8] Oksala A, Lehtinen A. Measurement of the velocity of sound in some parts of the eye. Acta Ophthalmologica. 1975:633-639

[9] Jansson F. Measurement of intraocular distances by ultrasound and comparison between optical and ultrasonic determinations of the depth of the anterior chamber. Acta Ophthalmologica. 1963;**41**:25-61. DOI: 10.1111/j.1755-3768.1963.tb02420.x

[10] Coleman DJ, Carlin B. A new system for visual Axis measurements in the human eye using ultrasound. Archives of Ophthalmology. 1967;**77**:124-127. DOI: 10.1001/archopht.1967.00980020126027

[11] Sanders DR, Kraff MC. Improvement of intraocular lens power calculation using empirical data. American Intra-Ocular Implant Society Journal. 1980;**6**:263-267. DOI: 10.1016/S0146-2776(80)80075-9

[12] Doppler C. Ueber das farbige Licht der Doppelsteme und einer anderer Gestirne des Himmels. Prag K Bohm. 1842

[13] Kasai C, Namekawa K, Koyano A, Omoto R. Real-time two-dimensional blood flow imaging using an autocorrelation technique. IEEE Transactions on Sonics and Ultrasonics. 1985;**32**:458-464. DOI: 10.1109/T-SU.1985.31615

[14] Ciccone TJ, Grossman SA. Cardiac ultrasound. Emergency Medicine Clinics of North America. 2004;**22**:621-640. DOI: 10.1016/j.emc.2004.04.012

[15] Hein IA, O'Brien WD. A flexible blood flow phantom capable of independently producing constant and pulsatile flow with a predictable spatial flow profile for ultrasound flow measurement validations. IEEE Transactions on Biomedical Engineering. 1992;**39**:1111-1122. DOI: 10.1109/10.168687

[16] Ferrara KW, Algazi VR, Liu J. The effect of frequency dependent scattering and attenuation on the estimation of blood velocity using ultrasound. IEEE Transactions on Ultrasonics, Ferroelectrics, and Frequency Control. 1992;**39**:754-767. DOI: 10.1109/58.165561

[17] Martin PJ, Evans DH, Naylor AR, Bell PRF. Transcranial colour coded sonography as an aid to measurement of blood flow velocity in the basal cerebral arteries. Ultrasound in Medicine & Biology. 1993;**19**:711-716. DOI: 10.1016/0301-5629(93)90088-6

[18] Macsweeney JE, Cosgrove DO, Arenson J. Colour Doppler energy (power) mode ultrasound. Clinical Radiology. 1996;**51**:387-390. DOI: 10.1016/S0009-9260(96)80155-3

[19] Cosgrove DO, Kedar RP, Bamber JC, al-Murrani B, Davey JB, Fisher C, et al. Breast diseases: Color Doppler US in differential diagnosis. Radiology. 1993;**189**:99-104. DOI: 10.1148/radiology.189.1.8372225

[20] Guerriero S, Alcazar JL, Ajossa S, Galvan R, Laparte C, García-Manero M, et al. Transvaginal color Doppler imaging in the detection of ovarian cancer in a large study population. International Journal of Gynecological Cancer. 2010;**20**:781-786

[21] Emerson DS, Cartier MS, Altieri LA, Felker RE, Smith WC, Stovall TG, et al. Diagnostic efficacy of endovaginal color Doppler flow imaging in an ectopic pregnancy screening program. Radiology. 1992;**183**:413-420. DOI: 10.1148/radiology.183.2.1561342

[22] AbuRahma AF, Srivastava M, Stone PA, Mousa AY, Jain A, Dean LS, et al. Critical appraisal of the carotid duplex consensus criteria in the diagnosis of carotid artery stenosis. Journal of Vascular Surgery. 2011;**53**:53-60. DOI: 10.1016/j.jvs.2010.07.045

[23] Luo J, Yan Z, Jia Y, Luo R. Clinical analysis of 42 cases of ocular ischemic syndrome. Journal of Ophthalmology. 2018;**2018**:1-7. DOI: 10.1155/2018/2606147

[24] Mokbel TH, Shahin MM, El-Said EM, El-Ghaffar WMA. Potential diagnostic value of fluorescein angiography and color Doppler imaging in primary open angle glaucoma. European Journal of Ophthalmology. 2009;**19**:957-962. DOI: 10.1177/112067210901900610

[25] Yamamoto Y. Doppler examination of blood flow in the ocular fundus. Bibliotheca Ophthalmologica. 1975;**83**:32-40

[26] Dennis KJ, Dixon RD, Winsberg F, Ernest JT, Goldstick TK. Variability in measurement of central retinal artery velocity using color Doppler imaging. Journal of Ultrasound in Medicine. 1995;**14**:463-466

[27] Bronson NR. Development of a simple B-scan ultrasonoscope. Transactions of the American Ophthalmological Society. 1972;**70**:365-408

[28] Coleman DJ, Konig WF, Katz L. A hand-operated, ultrasound scan system for ophthalmic evaluation. American Journal of Ophthalmology. 1969;**68**:256-263. DOI: 10.1016/0002-9394(69)94068-9

[29] Foster FS, Pavlin CJ, Harasiewicz KA, Christopher DA, Turnbull DH. Advances in ultrasound biomicroscopy. Ultrasound in Medicine & Biology. 2000;**26**:1-27. DOI: 10.1016/S0301-5629(99)00096-4

[30] Baum G, Greenwood I. The application of ultrasonic locating techniques to ophthalmology. A.M.A. Archives of Ophthalmology. 1958;**60**:263. DOI: 10.1001/archopht.1958.00940080279015

[31] Coleman DJ, Lucas BC, Rondeau MJ, Chang S. Management of intraocular foreign bodies. Ophthalmology. 1987;**94**:1647-1653. DOI: 10.1016/S0161-6420(87)33239-7

[32] Bronson NR II. Management of intraocular foreign bodies.

American Journal of Ophthalmology. 1968;**66**:279-284. DOI: 10.1016/0002-9394(68)92075-8

[33] Coleman DJ, Jack RL, Franzen LA, Coleman J. Ultrasonography in ocular trauma. American Journal of Ophthalmology. 1978;**75**:279-288. DOI: 10.1016/S0002-9394(14)76689-9

[34] BAUM G, GREENWOOD I. Ultrasonography—An aid in orbital tumor diagnosis. Archives of Ophthalmology. 1960;**64**:180-194. DOI: 10.1001/archopht.1960.01840010182003

[35] Oksala A. Echogram in melanoma of the choroid. The British Journal of Ophthalmology. 1959;**43**:408-414

[36] Oksala A. Ultrasound diagnosis in intraocular melanoma. Annals of the New York Academy of Sciences. 1963;**100**:18-28. DOI: 10.1111/j.1749-6632.1963.tb57110.x

[37] Baum G. Ultrasonographic characteristics of malignant melanoma. Archives of Ophthalmology. 1967;**78**:12-15. DOI: 10.1001/archopht.1967.00980030014003

[38] Coleman DJ. Reliability of ocular and orbital diagnosis with B-scan ultrasound. 2. Orbital diagnosis. American Journal of Ophthalmology. 1972;**74**:704-718

[39] Coleman DJ. Reliability of ocular and orbital diagnosis with B-scan ultrasound; 1. Ocular diagnosis. American Journal of Ophthalmology. 1972;**73**:501-516. DOI: 10.1016/0002-9394(72)90002-5

[40] Coleman DJ, Silverman RH, Rondeau MJ, Lizzi FL. New perspectives: 3-D volume rendering of ocular tumors. Acta Ophthalmologica. 2009;**70**:22-22. DOI: 10.1111/j.1755-3768.1992.tb04918.x

[41] Silverman RH, Coleman DJ, Rondeau MJ, Woods SM, Lizzi FL. Measurement of ocular tumor volumes from serial, cross-sectional ultrasound scans. Retina. 1993;**13**:69-74

[42] Pavlin CJ. Ultrasound Biomicroscopy. Ophthalmology Rounds. Vol. 2. 2004

[43] Stuart Foster F, Pavlin CJ, Lockwood GR, Ryan LK, Harasiewicz KA, Berube L, et al. Principles and applications of ultrasound backscatter microscopy. IEEE Transactions on Ultrasonics, Ferroelectrics, and Frequency Control. 1993;**40**:608-617. DOI: 10.1109/58.238115

[44] Sherar MD, Foster FS. Ultrasound backscatter microscopy. In: IEEE 1988 Ultrason. Symp. Proceedings. Chicago: IEEE; 1988. pp. 959-966. DOI: 10.1109/ULTSYM.1988.49519

[45] Pavlin CJ, Sherar MD, Foster FS. Subsurface ultrasound microscopic imaging of the intact eye. Ophthalmology. 1990;**97**:244-250. DOI: 10.1016/S0161-6420(90)32598-8

[46] Reinstein DZ, Silverman RH, Raevsky T, Simoni GJ, Lloyd HO, Najafi DJ, et al. Arc-scanning very high-frequency digital ultrasound for 3D pachymetric mapping of the corneal epithelium and stroma in laser in situ keratomileusis. Journal of Refractive Surgery. 2001;**16**:414-430

[47] Coleman DJ, Fish SK. Presbyopia, accommodation, and the mature catenary. Ophthalmology. 2001;**108**:1544-1551. DOI: 10.1016/S0161-6420(01)00691-1

[48] Silverman RH, Lizzi FL, Ursea BG, Rondeau MJ, Eldeen NB, Kaliscz A, et al. High-resolution ultrasonic imaging and characterization of the ciliary body. Investigative Ophthalmology & Visual Science. 2001;**42**:885-894

[49] Pavlin CJ, McWhae JA, McGowan HD, Foster FS. Ultrasound

biomicroscopy of anterior segment tumors. Ophthalmology. 1992;**99**:1220-1228. DOI: 10.1016/S0161-6420(92)31820-2

[50] Varghese M, Ramappa R, Kamath S. Pseudotumor of Ciliary body. Case Reports in Ophthalmological Medicine. 2014;**2014**:1-3. DOI: 10.1155/2014/458683

[51] Velazquez-Martin JP, Krema H, Fulda E, Yücel YH, Simpson ER, Pavlin CJ. Ultrasound biomicroscopy of the ciliary body in ocular/oculodermal melanocytosis. American Journal of Ophthalmology. 2013;**155**:681-687.e2. DOI: 10.1016/J.AJO.2012.10.006

[52] Suwan Y, Jiamsawad S, Supakontanasan W, Teekhasaenee C. Hidden mechanisms beyond the pupillary block in acute angle closure: Ultrasound biomicroscopic study. Clinical & Experimental Ophthalmology. 2017;**45**:366-370. DOI: 10.1111/ceo.12867

[53] Fisher Y, Hanutsaha P, Tong S, Fenster A, Mazarin G, Mandava N. Three-dimensional ophthalmic contact B-scan ultrasonography of the posterior segment. Retina. 1998;**18**:251-256

[54] Cusumano A, Coleman DJ, Silverman RH, Reinstein DZ, Rondeau MJ, Ursea R, et al. Three-dimensional ultrasound imaging. Clinical applications. Ophthalmology. 1998;**105**:300-306

[55] Peyman GA, Ingram CP, Montilla LG, Witte RS. A high-resolution 3D ultrasonic system for rapid evaluation of the anterior and posterior segment. Ophthalmic Surgery, Lasers, and Imaging. 2012;**43**:143-151. DOI: 10.3928/15428877-20120105-01

[56] Susal AL, Gaynon MW, Walker JT. Linear Array multiple transducer ultrasonic examination of the eye. Ophthalmology. 1983;**90**:266-271. DOI: 10.1016/S0161-6420(83)34564-4

[57] Blaivas M, Theodoro D, Sierzenski PR. A study of bedside ocular ultrasonography in the emergency department. Academic Emergency Medicine. 2002;**9**:791-799

[58] Cannata JM, Williams JA, Zhou Q, Ritter TA, Shung KK. Development of a 35-MHz piezo-composite ultrasound array for medical imaging. IEEE Transactions on Ultrasonics, Ferroelectrics, and Frequency Control. 2006;**53**:224-236. DOI: 10.1109/TUFFC.2006.1588408

Section 4

Biochemical Techniques

Chapter 6

Paper-Based ELISA: A Novel Diagnostic Approach for Monitoring Aqueous Humour VEGF Level in Ocular Diseases

Yu-Ting Tsao, Wei-Hsuan Sung, Hung-Chi Chen, Min-Yen Hsu and Chao-Min Cheng

Abstract

We commonly diagnose ocular diseases via both morphological changes and symptoms. It is necessary to develop biochemically based assays for early or follow-up diagnosis of these diseases with a focus on robustness and ease of handling. To lay out a prospective path toward this goal, we describe and propose the use of ultrahigh sensitive paper-based ELISA (p-ELISA), which uses a treated piece of filter paper to monitor the activity of ocular diseases (i.e., detecting the vascular endothelial growth factor (VEGF) concentration in aqueous humour for proliferative diabetic retinopathy or age-related macular degeneration diagnosis). The advantages of p-ELISA include the following: (1) the capacity to directly measure biomarker concentrations in aqueous humour using only a tiny sample volume (as little as 2 μL); (2) significantly increased sensitivity compared to conventional ELISA (fg/mL levels); and (3) inexpensive materials and a short operation duration. P-ELISA is a novel point-of-care diagnostic tool with the significant potential to advance ophthalmological treatment guidelines by facilitating early detection and routinely monitoring therapeutic response.

Keywords: paper-based ELISA, VEGF, diagnosis, ocular disease, ophthalmology, aqueous humour

1. Introduction

Prevention, diagnosis and treatment are the core principles of modern medical care. Two of these principles, prevention and treatment, are inextricably linked to the third, precise diagnosis. Suitable early diagnostic criteria must be established on properly understanding the pathophysiology of a specific disease and how it impacts the human body. Precise diagnosis naturally leads to precise prevention and treatment. By developing current biotechnologically relevant technologies, medical practitioners will have increasingly adequate tools for precise diagnoses and suitable monitoring of treatment methodologies. Most ophthalmologists, however, still diagnose ocular diseases based primarily on structural and functional changes. In this chapter, we will discuss biochemically based diagnostic tools for ophthalmology. The introduction consists of two parts: (1) an introduction to current

 IntechOpen

biochemically based diagnostic tools and the clinical applications of ELISA and (2) a discussion on the importance of VEGF monitoring for several eye diseases. Following this, we will present an overview and details on paper-based ELISA (p-ELISA), a rapid, cost-effective, easy-to-handle, sensitive, and robust method for monitoring aqueous humour VEGF level in ocular diseases.

1.1 ELISA in clinical applications

Biochemically based diagnostic tools have been widely used for a variety of specific clinical disease diagnoses, prognoses, and the evaluation of treatment efficacy. We have used such tools to measure specific tumor biomarkers as part of a multiple cancer screening tool (e.g., PSA screening for the prostate cancer), and to monitor CRP level to evaluate patient inflammatory state [1]. The focus of such biochemically based diagnostic tools is quantification or qualification of a target substance in body fluids to assist medical practitioners with precise disease diagnosis or treatment status [2]. To distinguish specific substances from body fluids, researchers have used multiple strategies including, but not limited to, enzyme-catalyzed reactions [3], antibody/antigen interactions, spectrophotometry [4], and electrophoresis [5]. Enzyme-catalyzed reactions and antibody/antigen interactions are two of the most widely applied technologies among biochemically based diagnostic tools. In the enzyme-catalyzed reactions model, the specific binding capabilities of enzymes facilitate the measurement of enzyme catalytic activities as a means of quantifying or qualifying a target substrate [6]. Raabo and Therkildsen first applied this strategy to measure blood sugar using glucose oxidase (GOD) [3]. In the antibody/antigen interactions model, quantitative capacity is provided by the immunological affinity between an antibody and a specific substrate or antigen, one of which is immobilized in the solid phase while the other is distributed in the liquid phase. This method is widely used in clinical biochemistry (e.g., detection of human chorionic gonadotropin in a pregnancy test [7]). Such methods are linked to the development of the enzyme-linked immunosorbent assay (ELISA), first described by Engvall and Perlmann, who combined the specificity of antibody/antigen interactions with signal amplification via high-turnover catalytic enzymes to provide both high sensitivity and specificity [8]. ELISA is traditionally performed in a 96-well plastic plate. Current formats of ELISA typically include the direct type, indirect type, sandwich type, and competitive type, with procedural details for each described in the chapter references [9]. The clinical importance of ELISA is the capacity to detect trace amounts of a particular peptide or protein (also known as antigen or antibody in an ELISA kit) in a rapid and executable way. ELISA is widely used as a screening or diagnostic tool. It is used for infectious disease screening, as in the detection of human immunodeficiency virus antigen (HIV-Ag) for the diagnosis of acquired immune deficiency syndrome (AIDS) [10]. It is employed for toxicology as in the detection of organophosphate in wheat end products [11]. And it is used for allergen screening in the food industry [12]. Conventional ELISA requires volumes of approximately 200 μL for test completion. Unfortunately, fluid sources such as aqueous humour are limited, which rules out conventional ELISA methodology for ocular disease detection. A modified ELISA, p-ELISA for instance, that could use minute sample volumes would be an invaluable tool in such cases.

1.2 Importance of monitoring VEGF levels within the human eye

Measuring the concentrations of specific circulating substrates (e.g., vascular endothelial growth factor (VEGF)) in aqueous humour or vitreous humour can provide ophthalmologists with a relevant tool for evaluating ocular diseases. Elevation of the VEGF plays a critical role in the pathological angiogenesis of age-related macular degeneration (AMD) and diabetic retinopathy (DR) [13], the two leading causes of blindness in developed countries. AMD is a degenerative disease characterized by loss of central vision. Clinically, we can classify AMD into neovascular and non-neovascular types. DR is one of the major complications of type 1 and type 2 diabetes mellitus. Over 30 million people suffer from vision-threatening DR worldwide [14]. Overexpression of VEGF in neovascular AMD and DR leads to neovascularization and vascular leakage, which eventually results in retinal thickening and edema [13, 15]. Both of the diseases mentioned above are diagnosed by symptomatic and structural examination using an ophthalmoscope, fluorescein angiography (FA), or optical coherence tomography (OCT). Both can be treated with intravitreal injection of VEGF inhibitors (for neovascular AMD and DR). Injection of anti-VEGF agents has become one of the most effective treatments for neovascular AMD and DR [16, 17]. Pegaptanib, ranibizumab, bevacizumab and aflibercept are the currently available anti-VEGF agents. Although anti-VEGF therapy has saved many patients from visual loss, the cost of anti-VEGF therapy is relatively high and requires lifelong treatment (e.g., in neovascular AMD, the cost was about €22,818–37,926 per year for bevacizumab, ranibizumab, and aflibercept therapy [18]). Unfortunately, the efficacy of anti-VEGF therapy varies from person to person, which provokes controversy over treatment time schedules. Individualized therapy is frequently advocated but limited by deficient tools to precisely monitor the progression of the pathological angiogenesis in eyes. It is commonly known that elevation of VEGF appears before clinically detectable structural or functional changes [19]. Clearly then, easy detection of VEGF levels within the human eye can decidedly assist early diagnosis, severity assessment (as a quantitative tool), and drug-efficacy evaluation.

Both the blood-ocular barrier and insufficient quantities of aqueous humour have limited the possibilities for biochemically based diagnostic tools for ocular diseases. In most cases, an ophthalmologist can only diagnose and follow up on ocular diseases via examination of morphological changes of the eyes and symptoms analysis. Unfortunately, anatomical changes and functional visual loss are largely, though not completely, irreversible. Therefore, it is necessary to develop an early detection technique to diagnose and monitor ocular diseases before visual acuity loss, and such a technique must be capable of using only small sample amounts. We believe that p-ELISA is just such a tool. It can be used to monitor VEGF levels with minute sample amounts and is capable of ultrahigh sensitivity and specificity.

2. How do we apply p-ELISA to monitor VEGF levels in ocular diseases?

Although the vitreous humour occupies the majority of the space in the human eye (about 4 mL in an adult eye) and contacts directly to the retina, it is difficult to extract the vitreous humour as a diagnostic sample for retina evaluation for two reasons: (1) the vitreous humour is stagnant and not actively replenished and (2) the risk of vitreous hemorrhage and retinal detachment when extracting vitreous humour. Several studies have reported that cytokine level in aqueous humour is highly correlated with vitreous level and severity of AMD and DR [20, 21]. For this reason, extracting aqueous humour is a safer source of material for monitoring VEGF level. Aqueous humour is produced from the ciliary process at an average rate of 2.4 μL/min [22] and fills the anterior and the posterior chambers. The total volume of an adult's aqueous humour is about 250 μL. The maximum amount of aqueous humour that can be extracted from the anterior chamber at one time before potential chamber collapse is approximately 200 μL.

The conventional ELISA plate requires relatively large sample volumes per assay (50–200 μL) compared to p-ELISA. Both the tolerance and repeatability of each test are restricted by sample volume, so small volumes are obviously problematic. While sample volume can be magnified via dilution, sensitivity and specificity are consequently diminished [23]. Moreover, complicated incubating and blocking steps in conventional ELISA are time-consuming and tedious and lead to a decrease in sensitivity and specificity. Conventional ELISA requires modification to more practical sample volumes on the scale of microliters, and sensitivity and specificity must be preserved or amplified.

P-ELISA requires only a piece of filter paper, and can effectively be used with well volumes as low as 3 μL. The high surface-to-volume ratio of cellulose fibers in paper greatly reduces reaction time so that a diagnostic procedure can be completed within a single hour (compared to approximately 4 h for conventional ELISA). P-ELISA also relies on methodology that is different from the conventional ELISA sandwich model: it uses an indirect model. Instead of using Avastin, the more traditional monoclonal antibody, p-ELISA uses HRP-conjugated Avastin. The simplified protocol and high affinity between antigen/antibody gives rise to ultrahigh sensitivity and specificity (fg/mL levels). Furthermore, recording and analyzing p-ELISA results can be completed by using a commercial handheld cellphone camera and image-processing software. In this way, expensive ELISA plate readers are replaced by inexpensive and common technology that allows small-scale laboratories to perform ELISA analysis in an easy-to-handle and cost-effective manner.

2.1 Production of the paper plate

P-ELISA was first introduced in 2010 by Chao-Min Cheng [24] who used a 96-microzone paper plate instead of a traditional plastic well to perform ELISA. His first 96-microzone paper plate was made using filter paper processed by photolithography to generate hydrophobic barriers between each test zone. He found that three-dimensional (3D) structures of the cellulose fiber network in the test zones boosted the reaction rate and reduced the required, effective sample volume to only 3 μL. Photolithography allowed mass plate production but required expensive equipment and a complicated production process. A less costly and simpler procedure was subsequently found: inkjet printing [25]. Of the various inkjet printing methods, wax printing and screen printing were found to be the two best, and now most common, strategies to produce 96-microzone paper plates. Wax printing uses a commercial wax printer to create hydrophobic patterns on filter paper, and screen printing uses commercially available polymer solutions [26, 27]. Both of these two methods are flexible, inexpensive, and easy to use.

Wax printing is an easy to execute and effective process for forming test zones on paper. The nature of the paper substrate allows for the creation of hydrophilic test zones, and the wax, printed in circles, makes defined hydrophobic barriers. The result is a sheet of paper with small, defined wells arrayed in a format that mimics that of a 96-well plate. This 96-well-plate format was first designed on a computer using commercial software (white areas as the hydrophilic test zones and black areas as the hydrophobic barriers), and then printed on Whatman qualitative paper with a commercial wax printer (Xerox Phaser 8560DN). The wax-printed paper was then placed on a hotplate (135°C) to melt the printed wax enough to allow it to penetrate all the way from the printed side through to the opposite side of the paper [28]. Careful attention was paid to this melting process to avoid heating for too long, which would result in the wax spreading out too far from its originally printed shape. Typically this process took from 10 to 20 min, but visual observation always took precedence over total time if necessary. Alternatively to using a hotplate, an oven could be used for this process, in which case the melting process was shorter in length. Test zone creation was visually verified by observing whether or not the black wax appeared on the back side of the paper or by placing a drop of water on the paper to test the integrity of the printed hydrophobic area. While the format of the paper plate test zone was identical to that of a traditional, plastic 96-well plate for conventional ELISA (circles of 5 mm in diameter), each well or test zone required only 3 μL of solution to fill (see **Figure 1**). Although a smaller test zone would require less sample volume, we chose the conventional 96-well plate format to facilitate familiarity and a relationship to standard protocols used in conventional laboratories.

2.2 How to perform ELISA on the paper plate

To simplify the ELISA protocol, we used an indirect ELISA model instead of the conventional sandwich ELISA model. Our protocol comprised 5 steps as follows: (1) antigen immobilization within test zones; (2) blocking the test zones with buffer; (3) adding enzyme conjugated detection antibodies; (4) washing away unbound antibodies; and (5) adding substrates for a color-producing enzymatic reaction. Antigen immobilization was completed via application and physical adsorption, a process based on the non-specific interaction between the antigens and the paper fibers [29]. This step requires approximately 3 μL of solution and 10 min of drying under ambient conditions. Blocking the test zones with the blocking buffer prevented nonspecific antibody binding. This step also required approximately 3 μL of solution and 10 min of drying. Enzyme-conjugated detection antibodies were added to conjugate with the immobilized antigen. Incubation period was dependent on experimental design. Washing away the unbound antibodies was completed with a piece of blotting

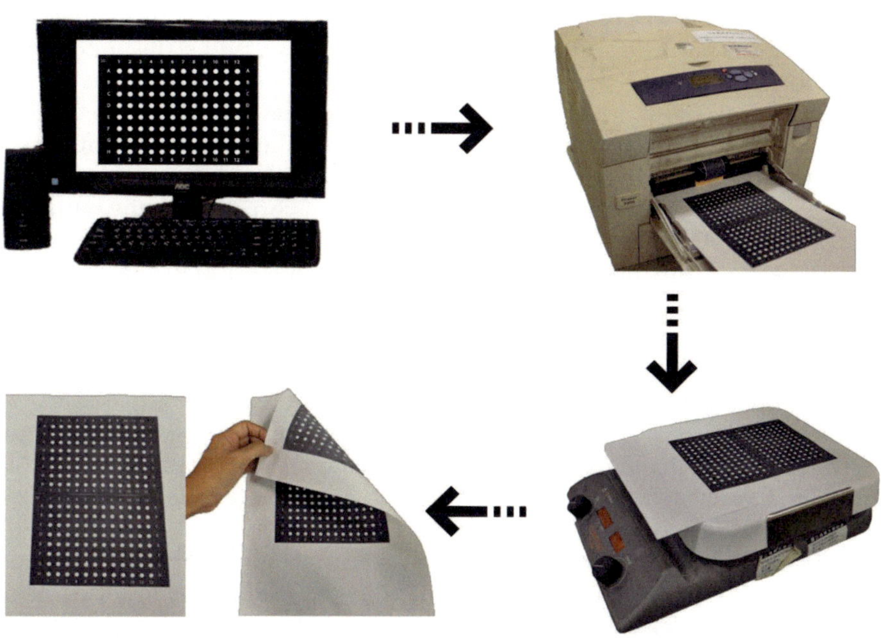

Figure 1.
The schematic of the paper plate production. The pattern of the paper plate was first designed using commercial software on a computer, and the pattern was printed onto Whatman qualitative paper using a wax printer. In the next step, the printed black wax was heated to melt it through the filter paper using a hot plate with the temperature set at approximately 135°C. This created defined hydrophobic barriers surround hydrophilic test zones. The pattern of the test zones should be clear on both side of the filter paper in the finished product.

paper placed beneath the paper plate to absorb the washing buffer, or the paper plate was shaken in a basin of washing buffer. The final step, adding substrates to initiate a color-producing enzymatic reaction with the conjugate enzyme, was performed immediately after the washing step. Total processing time for this colorimetric reaction varied from case to case, and some conditions, such as humidity and ambient temperature, affected evaporation rate, so controlling such variables is important for reducing experimental error. Following chemical processing, colorimetric results can be conveniently recorded using a desktop scanner or a commercial cellphone camera and then analyzed via software using a linear red-green-blue (RGB) system. Although a desktop scanner is the most commonly used analytical device for paper-based diagnostic tools due to its high sensitivity, the cellphone camera and application model has gained significant popularity due to its portability, convenience, and cost efficiency. An image interpretation application (e.g., Petgeia) can be used to analyze the colorimetric reaction. Moreover, several recent papers have shown that cellphone camera analytical results are comparable to those from a desktop scanner [30, 31]. Combining the convenience of using a simple paper substrate with a lightweight cellphone camera and application dramatically increases the practicality of such an approach for effective, real-time, point-of-care (POC) diagnostics that can significantly impact health outcomes for a number of people, especially those in resource-poor environments.

2.3 Protocol from aqueous humour extraction to aqueous VEGF level detection

We can now more easily relate the p-ELISA process to our real-life protocol for detecting VEGF levels in aqueous humour. The aqueous humour extraction was performed under a normal and proper process. All the patients were examined by the slit lamp first to evaluate the condition of anterior chamber, and the anterior chamber paracentesis was then performed by the following step: the patient was placed in a supine position and all the procedure was done under the microscope. Local anesthesia was given by dripping 0.5% proparacaine hydrochloride two to three times with an interval of 5 min. The surgical field was spread by the lid speculum and the eyeball was fixed at the limbus opposite to the paracentesis site. First ocular surface was disinfected by diluted beta-iodine solution for 5 min. Then, a 27 gauge needle was inserted through the paralimbal cornea carefully with the tip overlying and parallel to the iris. The bevel of the needle should be placed forward and carefully avoid hurting the lens. A volume of about 50–100 μL aqueous humour was extracted and put into storage for further analysis. 50–100 μL aqueous humour would be sufficient for detecting the VEGF level by repeating 20 wells in p-ELISA model, which required only 2 μL samples for analysis in each well. After sampling, prophylactic antibiotic drop and ointment were given. The whole procedure took less than 10 min to complete. For detecting the VEGF levels in aqueous humour, first the VEGF concentration calibration curve was produced by adding varying VEGF concentrations from a commercially available VEGF kit into a row of test zones. These concentrations ranged from 10^{-14} g/mL to 10^{-6} g/mL (n = 8) (**Figure 2**) [32]. The calibration curve was calculated using the Hill equation and the coefficient of determination (R^2) was found to be 0.9938. The resulting color intensity of different VEGF concentrations has an approximately linear relationship without considering the blank value [33]. When testing aqueous humour, we reduced the requisite sample volume from 3 to 2 μL due to the limited volumes available. After adding 2 μL of patient aqueous humour into several test zones, we allowed the sample to dry for 10 min. We then added 2 μL 1% BSA blocking buffer into the test zones and waited another 10 min for drying. In the next step, 5 μL of 0.8 mg/mL horseradish peroxidase (HRP)-conjugated Avastin was added as the

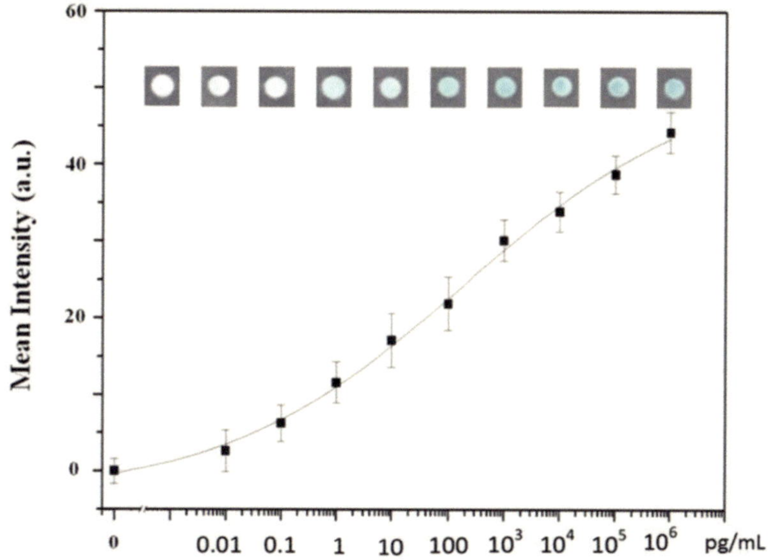

Figure 2.
The calibration curve of the of the commercially provided VEGF (kit form) using p-ELISA [34]. Eight different concentrations of commercial VEGF ranging from 10^{-14} g/mL to 10^{-6} g/mL were used. The calibration curve was calculated using the Hill equation, and the coefficient of determination (R^2) is 0.9938.

antibody, and the plates were incubated for 10 min to allow for conjugation with the immobilized VEGF. We then added 2.5 μL of streptavidin to enhance the colorimetric signal. After washing away the excess antibody with washing buffer, a 2 μL solution of 3,3′,5,5′-tetramethylbenzidine (TMB) + H_2O_2 was added into the test zones. This facilitated the enzyme substrate-driven colorimetric reaction with the HRP-conjugated Avistin. Resulting colorimetric output signals were dynamically recorded using a cellphone camera (from HTC Inc., Taiwan). For comparison, colorimetric results were also scanned using a commercial desktop scanner (EPSON; No.:GT-10000+). All images taken by these two optical recording approaches were then analyzed with image processing software (Adobe, Photoshop CS5), in order to compare the differences from each approach. This process was used to refine the more convenient cellphone-based recording system [33]. All procedures are performed in a laminar flow hood to prevent environmental bias and took less than 1 h to complete. The total equipment required in this protocol included several filter papers, a commercial wax printer, an oven, a pipetman, a commercial cellphone, and a desktop scanner, each of which are accessible and cost-effective. In addition to these efficiencies, the requirement of tiny sample volumes contributed to a reduction in overall cost for each test compared to conventional techniques.

The sensitivity of our p-ELISA to detect VEGF in a buffer system was ~33.7 fg/mL, which was outstanding for protein-detection technology and 150 times more sensitive than conventional ELISA (~5 pg/mL). The ultrahigh sensitivity of this new assay was attributed to several advantageous protocol features. First, we modified and prepared the antibody from human recombinant VEGF-A antibody to HRP-conjugated Avastin, and Avastin was the therapeutic antibody for VEGF, which carried high specificity toward VEGF. This therapeutic-based monoclonal antibody helped streamline the protocol with upgraded specificity. The HRP-conjugated Avastin was made following the protocol provided in an EasyLink HRP Conjugation Kit as described in detail in our reference information [33]. Secondly, we deviated from the conventional sandwich ELISA protocol to use an indirect ELISA protocol, which simplified the complicated blocking and washing steps. Lastly, we replaced the alkaline phosphate protocol for our colorimetric response with HRP (colorless to blue, instead of purple), allowing us to obtain the stronger output signals. The comparison between p-ELISA and conventional ELISA protocol for detecting aqueous humour VEGF levels is demonstrated in **Table 1**.

2.4 Clinical application of p-ELISA to detect VEGF levels in ophthalmological patients

In our previous study, we quantified aqueous humour VEGF levels in patients with several ocular diseases using p-ELISA. The mean VEGF levels detected in 13 senile cataract patients was 14.4 ± 8.5 pg/mL (mean ± SD), in 14 patients with proliferative DR (PDR), it was 740.1 ± 267.7 pg/mL, in 17 patients with AMD, it was 383 ± 155.5 pg/mL, and in 10 patients with retinal vein occlusion (RVO), it was 219.4 ± 92.1 pg/mL respectively [33]. In one study using conventional ELISA, Jian-Ping Tong reported that the mean VEGF levels from 10 senile cataract patients was 108.3 ± 72.3 (mean ± SD) pg/mL, while in 12 patients with choroidal neovascularization due to AMD it was 668.9 ± 340.0 pg/mL [20]. Similarly using conventional ELISA, Hideharu Funatsu reported mean VEGF levels of 26 patients with PDR as 376.5 ± 187.8 [21], and H Noma reported mean VEGF levels from 24 patients with branch RVO as 299.1pg/mL [34]. The pathogenesis of senile cataracts is rooted in degenerative effects on lens structure, which is different from the pathological angiogenesis of PDR, AMD, and RVO. Therefore, patients with senile cataract would be a good control group for our experiment. As we can see from the results mentioned above, both the p-ELISA and conventional ELISA showed considerable disparity in VEGF levels between patients with senile cataract and patients with PDR, AMD, or RVO (the levels of VEGF were low in the senile cataract group and high in PDR, AMD, or RVO groups). The aqueous VEGF levels measured by

	P-ELISA for VEGF		Conventional ELISA for VEGF	
Equipment	Paper plate Desktop scanner Smartphone camera		Plastic plate Plate readout	
Antigen/primary antibody	VEGF/HRP-conjugated avastin		VEGF/human recombinant VEGF-A antibody	
Secondary antibody	None		HRP conjugate	
Cost for equipment	100 USD		20,000 USD	
Dilution	No		Yes	
Detection sensitivity	0.03 pg		18.75 pg/mL	
Detection range	0.01–100,000 pg/mL		31.25–2000 pg/mL	
Reagent/duration	**Volume (μL)**	**Time (mins)**	**Volume (μL)**	**Time (mins)**
(1) Immobilize VEGF	2	7	70	120
(2) Blocking	2	7	100	30
(3) Antibody	7.5	20	30	60
(4) Colorimetric reaction (add TMB+ H_2O_2)	2	10	100	3
Total per zone	13.5	44	300	213
Total sample volume require per test	40 (repeat 20 wells)		9600 (total 96 wells)	

Table 1.
A comparison between conventional ELISA and p-ELISA in the detection of VEGF levels.

p-ELISA were comparable to those from conventional ELISA, supporting the idea that pathological angiogenesis can be adequately diagnosed using p-ELISA. Further case studies with greater sample numbers are necessary to confirm this.

In another one of our previous studies, we used p-ELISA to detect aqueous humour VEGF levels before and after intravitreal injection (IVI) of anti-VEGF antibodies.

The results showed that the mean VEGF levels in 16 patients with neovascular AMD, myopic neovascularization, or polypoidal choroidal vasculopathy were 545.71 ± 810.29 pg/mL (mean ± SD) before IVI of anti-VEGF antibodies. After IVI of anti-VEGF antibodies, the mean VEGF levels became 0.072–0.131 pg/mL (N = 15) within 5 weeks and 163.06 ± 367.06 pg/mL (N = 15) after 5 weeks. We also evaluated the efficacy of the ranibizumab and bevacizumab by detecting VEGF levels via p-ELISA and found that 50% of patients (6/12) that took ranibizumab demonstrated earlier VEGF elevation within 49 days compared to 11.11% (2/18) in patients that took bevacizumab (p = 0.0342) [32]. The minimal sample volume requirement and ultrahigh sensitivity of p-ELISA allowed us to monitor VEGF levels closely. Using this approach, ophthalmologists could prescribe personalized VEGF inhibitor treatment schedules for their patients. In addition, the delicate data output of p-ELISA could also assist clinicians and pharmaceutical companies to evaluate the effects of anti-VEGF antibodies. In summary, using p-ELISA to monitor aqueous VEGF level can be a useful tool to assist diagnosis of several ocular diseases, evaluate treatment efficacy of anti-VEGF treatment, and promote the development of new drugs.

Although the IVI of anti-VEGF antibodies has become one of the most powerful treatment strategies for patients with pathological angiogenesis in eye diseases, there are still many limitations to the clinical application of VEGF inhibitors:
(1) drug efficacy varies from person to person; (2) the adverse effects of IVI of VEGF antibiotics include post-injection endophthalmitis [35, 36], uveitis, rhegmatogenous retinal detachment, vitreous hemorrhage [36, 37], and the risk for sustained intraocular pressure elevation [36, 38]; and (3) the potential of systemic adverse events such as an increase in bleeding tendency [36]. Therefore, a good procedure for monitoring VEGF levels within the human eye would be beneficial to patients who receive VEGF inhibition therapy. In patients with good response to anti-VEGF therapies, a clinical ophthalmologist can decrease the frequency of VEGF inhibitor injections based on scheduled VEGF level monitoring by p-ELISA. Decreasing the frequency of IVI of VEGF antibiotics not only saves unnecessary medical expenses for patients, it spares the patients from the risk of therapeutic complications. For those patients with poor response to anti-VEGF therapies, early detection of elevated VEGF via ultrasensitive p-ELISA can alert a clinical ophthalmologist to increase treatment frequency or change the therapeutic approach. Because elevations in VEGF level appear earlier than morphological changes or visual acuity changes, monitoring VEGF levels can provide helpful early detection of disease and further prevent undesirable vision loss in those afflicted [39] (**Figure 3**). In addition to being ultrasensitive, p-ELISA for VEGF level detection takes only a short time (<1 h) compared to conventional ELISA (4–5 h). In a conventional outpatient clinical setting, aqueous humour extraction for VEGF level detection requires an initial visit, time-consuming testing, and a follow-up visit to discuss possible treatment options. With p-ELISA, a patient could be examined and receive results within an hour, hastening and increasing the efficacy of possible treatment (schematically described in **Figure 4**). Using p-ELISA for diagnosis as well as follow-up monitoring provides a more effective and less costly means of caring for patients without sophisticated laboratories and expensive ELISA readers. It offers a truly viable POC device that can be used in rural areas, in the developing world, and in emergency or resource-poor environments in ways that may revolutionize existing ocular disease diagnosis and treatment.

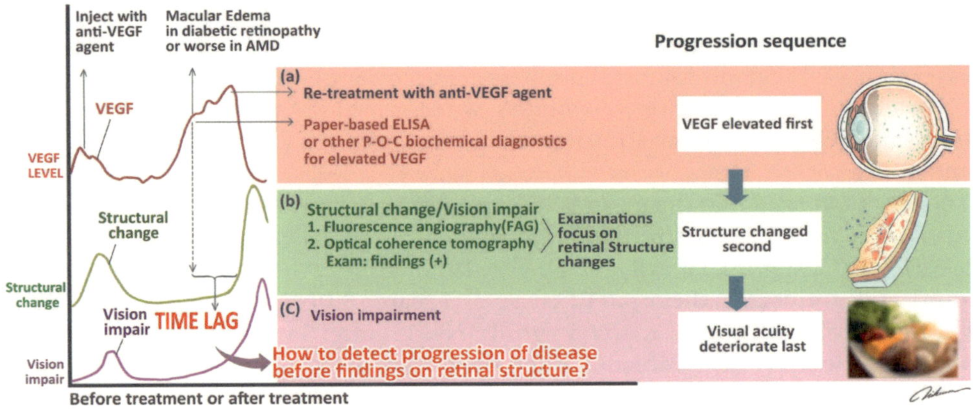

Figure 3.
The correlation between elevated VEGF, structural change, and vision impairment in patients receiving anti-VEGF therapy [39]. The Y coordinates represent VEGF levels, the structural changes, and vision impairment. The X coordinates represent the time sequence after the injection of anti-VEGF agent. Once the effects of the anti-VEGF agent began to wear off, VEGF levels initially elevated, leading to pathological angiogenesis, retinal structural changes, and vision impairment. Using an ultra-sensitive device such as p-ELISA to detect elevated VEGF levels would reduce the likelihood of structural changes and vision impairment. (a) P-ELISA or other POC diagnostics can detect elevated VEGF levels in the first disease progression sequence. (b) The structural changes could be noticed by FAG or OCT after a time lag of approximately 16 days following initial VEGF elevation. (c) Vision impairment would follow soon after the structural changes occurred.

2.5 The future prospects of paper-based ELISA

P-ELISA, first developed by the Whitesides Research Group at Harvard University to detect IgG and HIV antigen in serum, has become a useful diagnostic tool in many medical fields including the diagnosis of infectious disease (e.g., HIV, *E. coli*, and dengue fever [24, 28, 40]), the detection of autoimmune antibodies (e.g., anti-noncollagenous 16A (NC16A) in patients with bullous pemphigoid [41]), potential tumor marker assessment [42] and human cognitive performance determination (e.g., detecting specific neuropeptides such as neuropeptide Y following traumatic brain injuries and post-traumatic stress disorder [43]). We first used p-ELISA in the ophthalmological field to detect VEGF levels in aqueous humour and had good results in both disease diagnosis and treatment followed-up. P-ELISA is uniquely posed to meet the needs of eye disease diagnosis because it requires only tiny sample amounts to provide ultrahigh sensitive results. It is foreseeable that p-ELISA will take its place among commonly practiced approaches for diagnosing and treating ocular diseases. There are, in fact a great many detectable cytokines and growth factors in aqueous humour besides VEGF including tumor necrosis factor (TNF)-α, interleukin (IL)-2, -4, -5, -6, -8, -10, serum amyloid A (SAA), and migration inhibitory factor (MIF), and p-ELISA may ultimately be useful for detecting each of them. The elevation or depression of each of these markers is associated with ocular disease states [44–47]. It is worth noting that could the capacity to analyze a host of biomarkers with only tiny amounts (2 μL) of aqueous humour could lead to a comprehensive optical health examination that goes beyond and is more impactful than existing morphological and functional examinations.

As bright as the future is for this novel diagnostic technology, there are still existing limitations. Aqueous humour sampling is invasive, and low volume extraction does not eliminate risks of infection, hyphema, or lens capsule rupture. A less invasive strategy for evaluating ocular diseases would be ideal. We do know that tears carry a number of cytokines that are highly correlated with corneal and conjunctival disease. Elevation of IL-6, IL-8, and VEGF appears

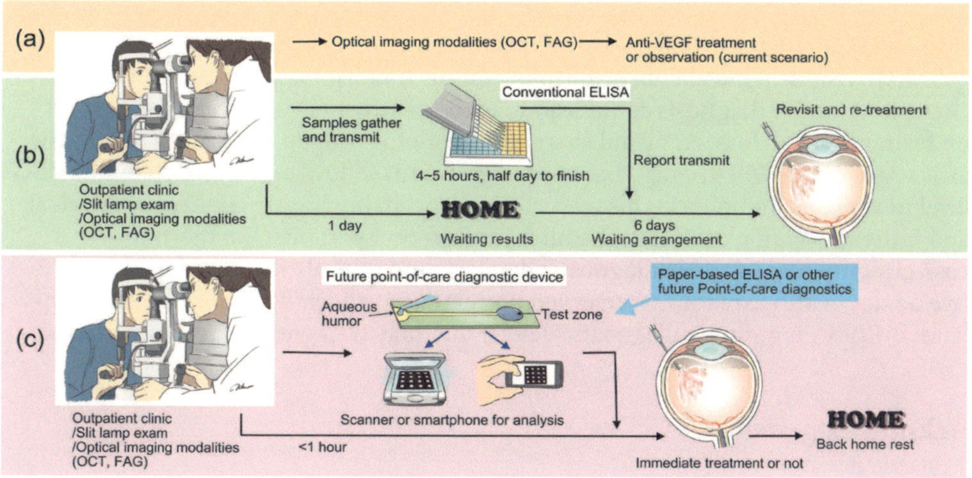

Figure 4.
The 3 different outpatient clinic scenarios for the follow-up examination of the patients receiving anti-VEGF treatment [39]. (a) Optical imaging modalities: the patient receives the optical imaging test only to determine whether to receive anti-VEGF treatment or observation. (b) Optical imaging + conventional ELISA VEGF level test: the patient receives the optical imaging test and extraction of aqueous humour occurs at the first visit. Because the conventional ELISA requires 4–5 hours to finish, the patient must arrange another appointment with the doctor to see the reports and decide whether to receive the anti-VEGF treatment. The next visit is usually one week later. This modality provides more information but has the risk of delaying treatment. (c) Optical imaging + p-ELISA VEGF level test: the patient receives the aqueous humour extraction, sees the testing reports, and decides whether to receive the treatments immediately within one visit. The short testing time of p-ELISA (<1 hr) allows the patient to obtain timely and proper treatment.

in patients with corneal neovascularization [48]. Elevation of inflammatory cytokines (IL-1β, IL-6, INF-γ, and TNF-α) indicates inflammation from ocular surface diseases [49, 50]. Detection of the trace amounts of biomarkers in tears by using ultra-sensitive p-ELISA is a direction for further investigation. P-ELISA has greatly simplified the complicated steps of conventional ELISA and eliminated the need for expensive equipment, but the process still requires professional medical technologists and simple laboratories for analyzing results, at least until cellphone camera applications become more developed. The properties of the p-ELISA as a lab-on-paper device make it a promising future POC device. Further modifying p-ELISA devices from an ophthalmologist-friendly diagnostic tool to a patient-friendly POC device remains a challenge. Development of an in situ device for ophthalmological analysis would provide considerable healthcare impact in developing countries with limited resources and alleviate the currently unbalanced ophthalmologist to patient ratio. This paper-based diagnostic tool is easy to handle, fast, sensitive, and requires only small samples and simple equipment to quantity specific biomarkers. P-ELISA has the potential to provide impactful benefit in the evaluation of ocular diseases and improve ocular health in real world.

3. Conclusions

In this chapter, we described how paper-based ELISA (p-ELISA) was robust, user-friendly, and required only small sample amounts (e.g., 2 μL of aqueous humour to measure VEGF) to return results that demonstrated very high sensitivity (~33.7 fg/mL). Detection of aqueous humour VEGF level via p-ELISA provides not only early diagnosis of ocular diseases with pathological angiogenesis (e.g., PDR,

AMD, and RVO), but assists in outlining accurate disease treatment. In regards to its effect on ocular disease diagnosis and treatment, p-ELISA can provide precise and quantitative biochemical data prior to the onset of morphological and functional changes. An early diagnosis could lead to early treatments and save patients from undesirable visual loss. As an aid to treatment monitoring, p-ELISA can record the efficacy of anti-VEGF therapy based on continuous follow-up measurement of VEGF level in aqueous humour. In this way, clinical ophthalmologists could provide ideal and individualized treatment schedules for different patients. Furthermore, this cost-effective and portable diagnostic device could provide far reaching and effective ocular health care for underserved populations especially in developing countries. P-ELISA is a simple diagnostic device that may well widen our views on eyes.

Acknowledgements

The authors thank the Ministry of Science and Technology of Taiwan for financially supporting this research under Contract No. MOST 107-2628-E-007-001-MY3 and 105-2221-E-007-053-MY3 (to C.-M. Cheng).

Conflict of interest

We declare that there is no conflict of interest.

Author details

Yu-Ting Tsao[1], Wei-Hsuan Sung[1], Hung-Chi Chen[2], Min-Yen Hsu[3] and Chao-Min Cheng[4*]

1 School of Traditional Chinese Medicine, Chang Gung University College of Medicine, Taoyuan, Taiwan

2 Department of Ophthalmology, Chang Gung Memorial Hospital, Linkou, Taiwan

3 Department of Ophthalmology, Chung Shan Medical University Hospital, Taichung, Taiwan

4 Institute of Biomedical Engineering, National Tsing Hua University, Hsinchu, Taiwan

*Address all correspondence to: chaomin@mx.nthu.edu.tw

References

[1] Young B, Gleeson M, Cripps AW. C-reactive protein: A critical review. Pathology. 1991;**23**:118-124. DOI: 10.3109/00313029109060809

[2] Gaw A, Murphy MJ, Srivastava R, et al. Clinical Biochemistry: An Illustrated Colour Text. 5th ed. Churchill Livingstone: Elsevier; 2013. 2-3 p

[3] Raabo BE, Terkildsen TC. On the enzymatic determination of blood glucose. Scandinavian Journal of Clinical and Laboratory Investigation. 1960;**12**:402-407. DOI: 10.3109/00365516009065404

[4] Trumbo TA, Schultz E, Borland MG, et al. Applied spectrophotometry: Analysis of a biochemical mixture. Biochemistry and Molecular Biology Education. 2013;**41**:242-250. DOI: 10.1002/bmb.20694

[5] Andrews AT. Electrophoresis: Theory, techniques and biochemical and clinical applications. In: Monographs on Physical Biochemistry. 2nd ed. Oxford, England, UK: Oxford University Press; 1986

[6] Cooper GM. The Cell: A Molecular Approach. 2nd ed. Sunderland (MA): Sinauer Associates; 2000. The Central Role of Enzymes as Biological Catalysts

[7] Cole LA. Immunoassay of human chorionic gonadotropin, its free subunits, and metabolites. Clinical Chemistry. 1997;**43**:2233

[8] Engvall E, Perlmann P. Enzyme-linked immunosorbent assay (ELISA) quantitative assay of immunoglobulin G. Immunochemistry. 1971;**8**:871-874. DOI: 10.1016/0019-2791(71)90454-X

[9] Aydin S. A short history, principles, and types of ELISA, and our laboratory experience with peptide/protein analyses using ELISA. Peptides. 2015;**72**:4-15. DOI: 10.1016/j.peptides.2015.04.012

[10] Allain JP, Paul DA, Laurian Y, et al. Serological markers in early stages of human immunodeficiency virus infection in haemophiliacs. The Lancet. 1986;**328**:1233-1236. DOI: 10.1016/S0140-6736(86)92673-5

[11] Skerritt JH, Guihot SL, Hill AS, et al. Analysis of organophosphate, pyrethroid, and methoprene residues in wheat end products and milling fractions by immunoassay. Cereal Chemistry. 1996;**73**:605-612

[12] vanHengel AJ. Food allergen detection methods and the challenge to protect food-allergic consumers. Analytical and Bioanalytical Chemistry. 2007;**389**:111-118. DOI: 10.1007/s00216-007-1353-5

[13] Witmer AN, Vrensen GFJM, Van Noorden CJF. Vascular endothelial growth factors and angiogenesis in eye disease. Progress in Retinal and Eye Research. 2003;**22**:1-29. DOI: 10.1016/S1350-9462(02)00043-5

[14] Lee R, Wong TY, Sabanayagam C. Epidemiology of diabetic retinopathy, diabetic macular edema and related vision loss. Eye and Vision. 2015;**2**:17. DOI: 10.1186/s40662-015-0026-2

[15] Shams N, Ianchulev T. Role of vascular endothelial growth factor in ocular angiogenesis. Ophthalmology Clinics of North America. 2006;**19**:335-344. DOI: 10.1016/j.ohc.2006.05.005

[16] Kovach JL, Schwartz SG, Flynn HW, et al. Anti-VEGF treatment strategies for wet AMD. Journal of Ophthalmology. 2012;**2012**:7. DOI: 10.1155/2012/786870

[17] Simó R, Hernández C. Intravitreous anti-VEGF for diabetic retinopathy:

Hopes and fears for a new therapeutic strategy. Diabetologia. 2008;**51**:1574. DOI: 10.1007/s00125-008-0989-9

[18] vanAsten F, Michels CTJ, Hoyng CB, et al. The cost-effectiveness of bevacizumab, ranibizumab and aflibercept for the treatment of age-related macular degeneration—A cost-effectiveness analysis from a societal perspective. PLoS One. 2018;**13**:e0197670. DOI: 10.1371/journal.pone.0197670

[19] Muether PS, Hermann MM, Viebahn U, et al. Vascular endothelial growth factor in patients with exudative age-related macular degeneration treated with ranibizumab. Ophthalmology. 2012;**119**:2082-2086. DOI: 10.1016/j.ophtha.2012.07.041

[20] Tong JP, Chan WM, Liu DTL, et al. Aqueous humour levels of vascular endothelial growth factor and pigment epithelium-derived factor in polypoidal choroidal vasculopathy and choroidal neovascularization. American Journal of Ophthalmology. 2006;**141**:456-462. DOI: 10.1016/j.ajo.2005.10.012

[21] Funatsu H, Yamashita H, Noma H, et al. Aqueous humour levels of cytokines are related to vitreous levels and progression of diabetic retinopathy in diabetic patients. Graefe's Archive for Clinical and Experimental Ophthalmology. 2005;**243**:3-8. DOI: 10.1007/s00417-004-0950-7

[22] Goel M, Picciani RG, Lee RK, et al. Aqueous humour dynamics: A review. The Open Ophthalmology Journal. 2010;**4**:52. DOI: 10.2174/1874364101004010052

[23] Kumar S, Kumar Y, Malhotra DV, et al. Standardisation and comparison of serial dilution and single dilution enzyme linked immunosorbent assay (ELISA) using different antigenic preparations of the Babesia (Theileria) equi parasite. Veterinary Research. 2003;**34**:71-83. DOI: 10.1051/vetres:2002055

[24] Cheng CM, Martinez AW, Gong J, et al. Paper-based ELISA. AngewandteChemie International Edition. 2010;**49**:4771-4774. DOI: 10.1002/anie.201001005

[25] Abe K, Suzuki K, Citterio D. Inkjet-printed microfluidic multianalyte chemical sensing paper. Analytical Chemistry. 2008;**80**:6928-6934. DOI: 10.1021/ac800604v

[26] Carrilho E, Martinez AW, Whitesides GM. Understanding wax printing: A simple micropatterning process for paper-based microfluidics. Analytical Chemistry. 2009;**81**:7091-7095. DOI: 10.1021/ac901071p

[27] Sun JY, Cheng CM, Liao YC. Screen printed paper-based diagnostic devices with polymeric inks. Analytical Sciences. 2015;**31**:145-151. DOI: 10.2116/analsci.31.145

[28] Lo SJ, Yang SC, Yao DJ, et al. Molecular-level dengue fever diagnostic devices made out of paper. Lab on a Chip. 2013;**13**:2686-2692. DOI: 10.1039/C3LC50135C

[29] Nisnevitch M, Firer MA. The solid phase in affinity chromatography: Strategies for antibody attachment. Journal of Biochemical and Biophysical Methods. 2001;**49**:467-480. DOI: 10.1016/S0165-022X(01)00214-7

[30] Martinez AW, Phillips ST, Carrilho E, et al. Simple telemedicine for developing regions: Camera phones and paper-based microfluidic devices for real-time, off-site diagnosis. Analytical Chemistry. 2008;**80**:3699-3707. DOI: 10.1021/ac800112r

[31] Shen L, Hagen JA, Papautsky I. Point-of-care colorimetric detection with a smartphone. Lab on a

Chip. 2012;**12**:4240-4243. DOI: 10.1039/C2LC40741H

[32] Hsu MY, Hung YC, Hwang DK, et al. Detection of aqueous VEGF concentrations before and after intravitreal injection of anti-VEGF antibody using low-volume sampling paper-based ELISA. Scientific Reports. 2016;**6**:34631. DOI: 10.1038/srep34631

[33] Hsu MY, Yang CY, Hsu WH, et al. Monitoring the VEGF level in aqueous humour of patients with ophthalmological diseases via ultrahigh sensitive paper-based ELISA. Biomaterials. 2014;**35**:3729-3735. DOI: 10.1016/j.biomaterials.2014.01.030

[34] Noma H, Funatsu H, Yamasaki M, et al. Aqueous humour levels of cytokines are correlated to vitreous levels and severity of macular oedema in branch retinal vein occlusion. Eye. 2006;**22**:42. DOI: 10.1038/sj.eye.6702498

[35] Meredith TA, McCannel CA, Barr C, et al. Postinjection endophthalmitis in the comparison of age-related macular degeneration treatments trials (CATT). Ophthalmology. 2015;**122**:817-821. DOI: 10.1016/j.ophtha.2014.10.027

[36] Falavarjani KG, Nguyen QD. Adverse events and complications associated with intravitreal injection of anti-VEGF agents: A review of literature. Eye. 2013;**27**:787. DOI: 10.1038/eye.2013.107

[37] Tufail A, Patel PJ, Egan C, et al. Bevacizumab for neovascular age related macular degeneration (ABC Trial): Multicentrerandomised double masked study. BMJ. 2010;**340**:c2459. DOI: 10.1136/bmj.c2459

[38] Choi DY, Ortube MC, McCannel CA, et al. Sustained elevated intraocular pressures after intravitreal injection of bevacizumab, ranibizumab, and pegaptanib. Retina. 2011;**31**:1028-1035. DOI: 10.1097/IAE.0b013e318217ffde

[39] Hsu MY, Chen SJ, Chen KH, et al. Monitoring VEGF levels with low-volume sampling in major vision-threatening diseases: Age-related macular degeneration and diabetic retinopathy. Lab on a Chip. 2015;**15**:2357-2363. DOI: 10.1039/C4LC01052C

[40] Shih CM, Chang CL, Hsu MY, et al. Paper-based ELISA to rapidly detect *Escherichia coli*. Talanta. 2015;**145**:2-5. DOI: 10.1016/j.talanta.2015.07.051

[41] Hsu CK, Huang HY, Chen WR, et al. Paper-based ELISA for the detection of autoimmune antibodies in body fluid—The case of bullous pemphigoid. Analytical Chemistry. 2014;**86**:4605-4610. DOI: 10.1021/ac500835k

[42] Wang S, Ge L, Song X, et al. Paper-based chemiluminescence ELISA: Lab-on-paper based on chitosan modified paper device and wax-screen-printing. Biosensors and Bioelectronics. 2012;**31**:212-218. DOI: 10.1016/j.bios.2011.10.019

[43] Murdock RC, Shen L, Griffin DK, et al. Optimization of a paper-based ELISA for a human performance biomarker. Analytical Chemistry. 2013;**85**:11634-11642. DOI: 10.1021/ac403040a

[44] van Kooij B, Rothova A, Rijkers GT, et al. Distinct cytokine and chemokine profiles in the aqueous of patients with uveitis and cystoid macular edema. American Journal of Ophthalmology. 2006;**142**:192-194. DOI: 10.1016/j.ajo.2006.02.052

[45] Santos Lacomba M, Marcos Martín C, Gallardo Galera JM, et al. Aqueous humour and serum tumor necrosis factor-α in clinical uveitis. Ophthalmic Research. 2001;**33**:251-255. DOI: 10.1159/000055677

[46] Takai Y, Tanito M, Ohira A. Multiplex cytokine analysis of

aqueous humour in eyes with primary open-angle glaucoma, exfoliation glaucoma, and cataract. Investigative Ophthalmology & Visual Science. 2012;**53**:241-247. DOI: 10.1167/iovs.11-8434

[47] Takase H, Futagami Y, Yoshida T, et al. Cytokine profile in aqueous humour and sera of patients with infectious or noninfectious uveitis. Investigative Ophthalmology & Visual Science. 2006;**47**:1557-1561. DOI: 10.1167/iovs.05-0836

[48] Zakaria N, Van Grasdorff S, Wouters K, et al. Human tears reveal insights into corneal neovascularization. PLoS One. 2012;**7**:e36451. DOI: 10.1371/journal.pone.0036451

[49] Wei Y, Gadaria-Rathod N, Epstein S, et al. Tear cytokine profile as a noninvasive biomarker of inflammation for ocular surface diseases: Standard operating procedures. Investigative Ophthalmology & Visual Science. 2013;**54**:8327-8336. DOI: 10.1167/iovs.13-12132

[50] Yamaguchi T, Calvacanti BM, Cruzat A, et al. Correlation between human tear cytokine levels and cellular corneal changes in patients with bacterial keratitis by in vivo confocal microscopy. Investigative Ophthalmology & Visual Science. 2014;**55**:7457-7466. DOI: 10.1167/iovs.14-15411

Section 5

Innovative Diagnostic Tools for Ophthalmology in Low Income Countries

Chapter 7

Innovative Diagnostic Tools for Ophthalmology in Low-Income Countries

Jason Singh, Sami Kabbara, Mandi Conway, Gholam Peyman and Robin D. Ross

Abstract

Globally, there are almost 300 million people blind and visually impaired and over 90% live developing countries. The gross disparity in access to ophthalmologists limits the ability to accurately diagnose potentially blinding conditions like cataract, glaucoma, trachoma, uncorrected refractive error and limits timely initiation of medical and surgical treatment. Since 85% of blindness is preventable, bridging this chasm for care is even more critical in preventing needless blindness. Many low-income countries must rely on community health workers, physician assistants, and cataract surgeons for primary eye care. Ophthalmology in low-income countries (LIC) is further challenging due to complexities brought from tropical climates, frail electric grids, poor road and water infrastructure, limited diagnostic capability and limited treatment options. Vision 2020 set the goal of eliminating preventable blindness by 2020 despite formidable obstacles. Innovative technologies are emerging to test visual acuity, correct refractive error quickly and inexpensively, capture retinal images with portable tools, train cataract surgeons using simulators, capitalize on mHealth, access ophthalmic information remotely. These advancements are allowing nonspecialized ophthalmic practitioners to provide low-cost, high impact eye care in resource-limited regions around the world.

Keywords: Vision 2020, preventable blindness, smartphone photography, mHealth

1. Introduction

When refractive error and presbyopia are included, more than 1.6 billion people suffer from some form of visual impairment worldwide [1]. Unfortunately, the greatest burden of visual blindness and impairment falls to the poor who are living in LIC where access to resources and eye care providers is scarce. According to a published report in 2010, the leading causes of blindness (defined as visual acuity in the better eye less than 3/60) were cataracts (33% of total cases of blindness), uncorrected refractive error (21% of cases), and macular degeneration (7% of cases) [2]. The leading causes of moderate and severe vision impairment (defined as visual acuity in the better eye less than 6/18 but at least 3/60) were uncorrected refractive error (53% of cases), cataract (18%), and macular degeneration (3%). However, these causes varied widely by region. Avoidable vision loss, due to conditions such as uncorrected refractive error, cataract, etc., which are treatable, is still a major problem worldwide. It accounts for 85% of all cases of vision loss. The number of avoidable cases of blindness is also increasing over time. By 2020, there will be a projected 76 million blind individuals globally.

The prevalence of childhood blindness and vision impairment (CBVI) varies based on socioeconomic development. For example, in high-income counties (HIC), the prevalence of blindness is 0.3 per 1000 children, while in LICs it is 1.5 per 1000 children. The number of blind children is estimated to be 1.4 million, with up to three-quarters of the blind children living in the poor regions of Africa and Asia. Some of the major causes of blindness and visual impairment in children of LIC include vitamin A deficiency, rubella cataracts, corneal scarring from measles, the use of harmful toxic eye remedies and ophthalmia neonatorum [3]. Immunizations and vitamin A supplements are proven, cost-effective preventions.

Despite these challenges, significant technological innovations provide an optimistic view for ending preventable blindness. This chapter will discuss the innovative devices that are currently being tested and used in order to promote eye health worldwide and help achieve the goals set forth by Vision 2020. These include low-cost, portable means of detecting refractive error and imaging the fundus, self-refracting glasses that do not require an eye care specialist, simulators to teach cataract surgery more efficiently, artificial intelligence that diagnose disease, and portable auto-phoropters. Future studies to validate these new innovations will be an important field of research.

2. Vision 2020

In 1999, the World Health Organization (WHO) launched an initiative called Vision 2020: The right to sight [4]. The objective of the initiative was to eliminate avoidable causes of blindness around the world and prevent the projected increase of avoidable visual impairment cases worldwide. Since then more than 90 nongovernmental organizations, agencies, institutions, and corporations have pledged their support of this initiative. If successful, this would reduce the cases of blindness from 76 million to below 25 million. The program is based on several core principles: human resource development, infrastructure and technology development, disease control, advocacy, and collaboration among stakeholders in eye health.

A 2014 study assessed the progress of 21 sub-Saharan African (SSA) countries toward the specific goals placed by the Vision 2020 [5]. The results were not encouraging. First, the authors noted that it was exceedingly difficult to access information on human resources for eye health within the study population, a necessary set of data in order to assist Vision 2020 planning. Secondly, the study found that few of the 21 countries met the human resources goals for the 2011 benchmark: only five countries met the goal for the number of ophthalmologists/cataract surgeons, four countries for ophthalmic nurses, and only two countries for cataract surgical rates (cataract surgeries as a ratio of operations per million population per year). No country met the goal target for number of optometrists, even when other personnel who perform refraction were considered. Overall, sub-Saharan African met three-quarters of its target for number of ophthalmologists, but only one-quarter of its goal for the number of ophthalmic nurses. Thirdly, the study found significant geographic inequities with higher concentrations of human resources in urban cities, seemingly at the expense of rural areas. As a result, there is still significant progress to be made. Compounding these existing provider shortages are increasing clinical care needs due to infectious epidemics, such as Ebola and Zika, and noncommunicable diseases, diabetes and hypertension, which pose a different epidemic threat level by 2030.

3. Innovative technologies

3.1 Refractive error testing kits

Uncorrected refractive error is the most common cause of preventable visual impairment worldwide [6]. The measurement of refractive error typically requires an eyecare specialist, a limiting factor in the provision of eyeglasses in LICs. One study in rural India found that more than 65% of a population with high rates of refractive error correctable with glasses were not wearing them due to inadequate access [7]. While in the U.S., there is approximately one eyecare professional for every 5500 people, that figure is only one per 1 million in certain parts of Africa [8, 9]. Such disparity has negative implications on sustaining educational and occupational productivity of these affected communities. The annual loss in global GDP due to distance visual impairment caused by uncorrected refractive error was an estimated $202 billion in 2007. In this section, we review various new technological innovations that are able to measure refractive error in a mobile, low-cost manner with limited personnel.

The Portable Eye Examination Kit (PEEK) solutions are built on smartphone technology which includes visual acuity apps and hardware, PEEK Retina. The smartphone app, Peek Acuity Pro, allows users to go through a brief tutorial and then tests visual acuity through a gamelike environment using a tumbling E (https://mts.intechopen.com/download/index/process/335/authkey/4eb406caf486438fcbbf872a81061e61). Peek Acuity has been shown to be an accurate and validated method to quickly test visual acuity [10]. Readings can be obtained in Imperial (20/20), Metric (6/6) or LogMar (0) for clinical research. The measured visual acuity can be simulated with a split screen view of a classroom chalkboard on one side compared to 20/20 view on the opposite side. The PEEK Retina allows fundus photography of the optic nerve and macula using a smartphone hardware attachment (**Figures 1** and **2**).

A qualitative study [11] in the Nakuru district of Kenya accessed the usability and acceptability of PEEK for providing eye care. In a region with a lack of adequate eye care services, patients found the PEEK system highly practical, as it allowed health practitioners to visit them in their own rural areas. This is particularly significant in regions with poor infrastructure and roads that can make transportation difficult. The PEEK system was also able to save patient time, overcoming the challenge of taking time off work and losing potential income. In regions where

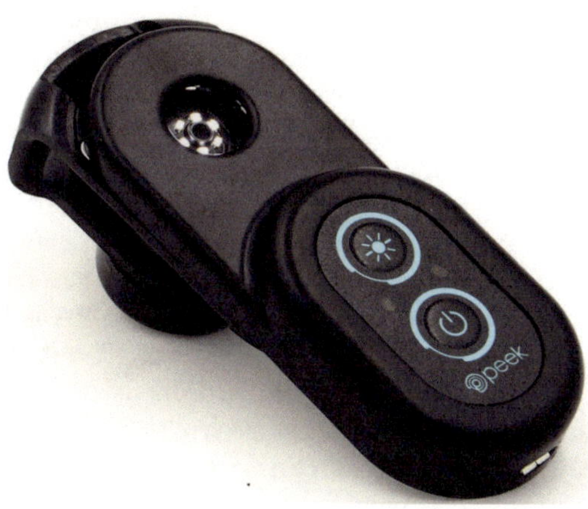

Figure 1.
The peek retina device.

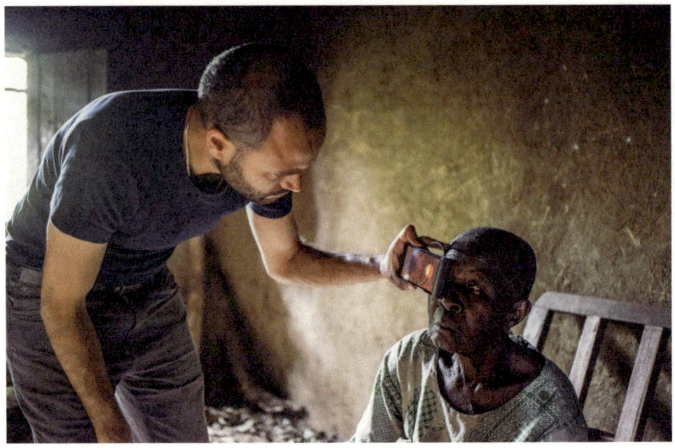

Figure 2.
Peek retina can be attached to a smartphone for portable fundal examinations.

eye problems are not perceived to be serious enough to warrant travel for care, barriers such as transportation become significant obstacles in providing eye care services. Patients and PEEK-trained healthcare workers appeared to have positive attitudes toward using mobile health technology, referring to it as "innovative" and "new." Many patients thought it to be efficient and cost-saving. Reasons for preferring PEEK were shorter exam times, simplicity, being seen at home, and increased ability to cover the population in need. However, some patients did prefer the traditional examination due to the ease of reading larger letters.

Another study [12] investigated whether a PEEK-based system could increase hospital follow-up for school aged children who were screened for visual impairment. Subjects in the experimental group determined to have visual impairment were shown their simulated sight on a smartphone and given a printout of this simulation. This simulation was then shared with the subjects' teachers and parents on a handout, which also included a written hospital referral letter. Parents in the experimental group were also sent regular SMS reminders to attend their follow-up appointment at the hospital. Compared to a control group which only received a referral letter without any simulation or SMS follow-up, the study found that visually impaired subjects in the PEEK group were significantly more likely to follow up at the hospital versus the control group with an odds ratio of 7.35 (95% CI 3.49–15.47). While the SMS reminders may have played a significant role in these results, future studies should analyze the effect of the simulation alone in increasing referral follow ups. However, one potential problem of increased screenings and referrals with PEEK or similar devices would be the inability of providers to handle the increased caseload. Nevertheless, PEEK have played a major role in addressing the shortage of vision care in underprivileged communities worldwide.

EyeNetra Inc. (Cambridge, MA) produces similar smartphone-based autorefractors for refractive error measurements (**Figure 3**). The autorefractor, NETRA, measures sphere, cylinder, axis, and pupillary distance in a virtual reality environment similar to that of PEEK. The age range for the NETRA is 10–65 years. The process takes 2 minutes and requires no power source. The company claims to be as accurate as autorefractors that cost $45,000, with its own product priced at $1290. Its system has an accuracy of 0.35D and comes with an extended battery for 2 days of testing without requiring a charge. It can withstand a drop from 1 m without breaking or losing accuracy, a convenient feature for users intending on traveling extensively with the device. EyeNetra also has a lensometer, called the Netrometer, that costs $975, and a phoropter, called the Netropter, which costs $699. The

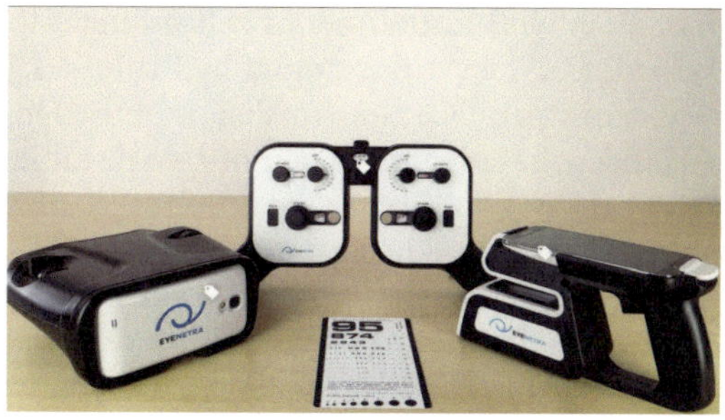

Figure 3.
The EyeNetra system includes an autorefractor, lensometer, and a phoropter (shown adjacent to a standard near card for size comparison).

combination of the three products can fit within a small suitcase to set up a mobile clinic virtually anywhere and provide all the tools needed to prescribe eyeglasses. The complete kit costs $2990. The EyeNetra products have been deployed in more than 90 countries worldwide.

In a study sponsored by EyeNetra, Inc., NETRA was compared with Zeiss iProfile Plus and subjective refraction on teenagers of age ranging from 14 to 18 years [13]. When NETRA was compared with subjective refraction, the average absolute difference in sphere was 0.48D, cylinder was 0.30D, and axis was 7.32°. One the other hand, when Zeiss iProfile Plus was compared with subjective refraction, the average absolute difference in sphere was 0.29D, cylinder was 0.45D, and axis was 11°.

Other handheld autorefractors include Retinomax 3, HAR 800/880, QuickSee, PlusOptix, Suresight, SVOne, WA Spot, and 2Win. Retinomax K-plus3, developed by Righton, is a handheld autorefractor and keratometer. It weighs around 1 kg and is able to perform keratometer and refraction measurements in around 0.34 seconds. Its battery life is around 80 minutes. The age range of Retinomax K-plus3 is 5–50 years old with a sphere range of −18.00D to +23.00D. However, pricing can be an issue to certain eyecare providers as it is priced around USD 11,000. HAR-800/880, developed by MOPTIM Imaging Technique Co. (Shenzhen, China), is a portable autorefractor that weighs approximately 0.9 kg with a battery life of 6 hours. The intended patient age range is 10–65 years with the sphere range of −6.0D to +8.0D. HAR-800/880 is priced at USD 4300. QuickSee is an autorefractor developed by PlenOptika (Massachusetts, USA). It is priced around USD 6000. It weighs around 1 kg and is able to perform refraction in 10 seconds. Its intended patient age is 5–85 years with spherical range of −10D to +10D. The battery life is approximately 6–8 hours. QuickSee has already been compared to experienced refractionists in rural south India, which found only small benefit to using subjective refraction over autorefraction [14]. More than half of the patients reported either no preference or preferred the autorefractor over subjective refraction. SVOne, developed by Smart Vision Labs (New York, NY), is a handheld autorefractor that weighs around 0.5 kg and costs USD 10,000. The intended patient age is 5–50 years with spherical range of −14D to +14D. It has been tested in LICs like Boliva by the Friends of Bolivia Foundation, Inc. PlusOptix, WA Spot and 2Win are handheld autorefractors intended for patients under the age of eight. The price of these autorefractors range from USD 6000–8000.

3.2 Self-adjustable glasses

Self-adjustable glasses are a recent innovation in the realm of optics and refractive error treatment. Also known as self-refraction, self-adjustable glasses look like any other set of glasses. A well-known set of self-adjustable glasses, Adspecs (Adaptive Eyecare, Oxford, UK), were developed by Professor Joshua Silver in conjunction with Dow Corning and Center for Vision in the Developing World (CVDW). Adspecs use lenses that are composed of two flexible membranes capable of moving inward or outward depending on the amount of silicone solution contained between them (**Figure 4**). The amount of the solution can be altered by the user using a syringe which moves fluid into or out of each lens. When fluid is pumped in, the curvature and power of the lens is increased. The user adjusts the amount of fluid until proper vision is attained, thereby correcting myopia or hyperopia. Another type of self-refracting glasses, USee, work by using pop-in best-sphere lenses (**Figure 5**). On the other hand, a design known as Alvarez optics uses two lens systems that move relative to each other in a spectacle frame, causing changes in lens power. Types of glasses that use this design are the FocusSpecs, Adlens, and Eyejusters.

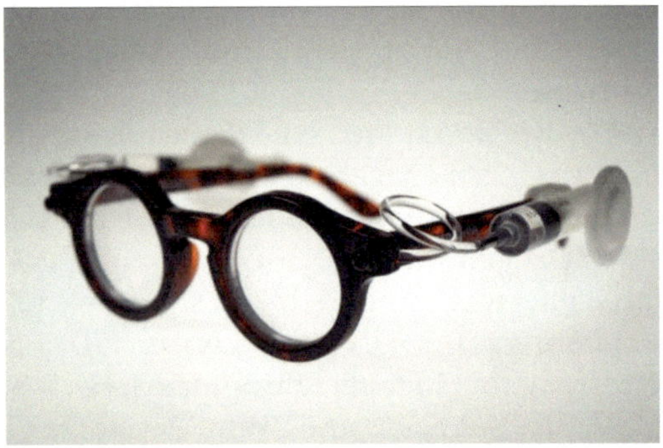

Figure 4.
Adspecs glasses can quickly adjust refractive power based on the amount of silicone solution injected into the spectacles.

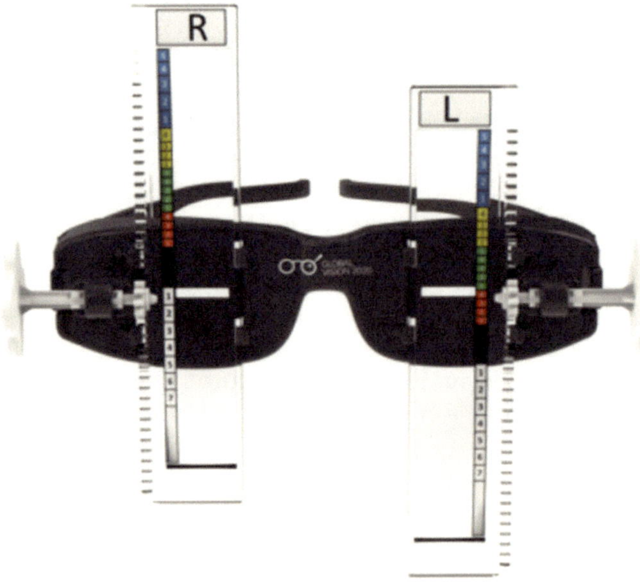

Figure 5.
USee glasses adjust refractive power by using pop-in, best-sphere lenses.

The first iteration of the Adspecs glasses cost between $18 and 19 to produce and the price has been decreasing ever since [15]. Studies have shown that Adspecs could lead to excellent visual outcomes [16]. A study in rural China found that, while visual acuity was slightly worse with self-refraction versus automated or subjective refraction, acuity was still very good [17]. Moreover, a study in urban Chinese children similarly found good visual acuity with self-refraction, but greater spherical and cylindrical refractive errors were associated with less accurate results as the range for the devices are limited to −6 to +6 D. Additionally, the adjustable glasses could not correct astigmatism [18]. Adjustable glasses are easy to use as is evident in a study that looked at users of USee which found positive results in 95% of the users [19].

Concerns regarding self-refracting glasses include the cosmetic appearance, the limited range of correction, inability to correct astigmatism, and compliance with international standards. The Adspecs have the additional limitation that once the glasses are self-adjusted and the power is fixed, they are unalterable. Despite being less expensive than traditional spectacles, cost is still a major barrier to self-adjustable glasses. One study in East Timor showed that nearly half the population was not willing to pay more than $1 for a pair of glasses [20]. Thus further reductions in cost are paramount for making the glasses affordable to worldwide.

3.3 Smartphone applications

Many iOS and Android applications exist for use in eye care and represent another low-cost tool for providing eye care globally. They generally fall within three categories: patient assessment tools, patient education tools, and health-care reference tools [21]. Many of the applications have redundant functions. For example, countless applications are available to visual acuity. Validation in a low-income setting is critical to compare applications to gold standard methods which can rely on calibration, optotype, distance, lamination and cultural settings. Applications also differ in the number of features they offer, price point, quality of user interface, and, perhaps most importantly, whether they continue to be supported by the developer over time. An analysis of the iTunes store shows that multiple applications from previous reviews [21] are no longer supported by the developers. This demonstrates that ophthalmic applications are part of a dynamic market that is ever-changing, with new applications entering the market each year with older applications exiting the marketplace. This presents the need for users to focus on applications that continue to be upgraded with subsequent iOS and Android updates.

The Eye Handbook (Cloud Nine Development) is the smartphone application currently most highly recommended by the authors for use in LICs (**Figure 6**). It is the most popular and successful application available in eye care [22]. As of 2018, it had over 2 million downloads. The Eye Handbook (EHB) is being used worldwide with 50% of downloads in North America, 20% in Europe, and 10% in each Asia and Australia [23]. While there are surely multiple equality applications that currently exist, the EHB has several significant advantages. First, it has shown to stand the test of time. EHB was developed in 2010 and continues to be supported and upgraded by the developers. Second, EHB is a free application thus making it ideal for use in LICs. Many other applications with similar features charge several dollars (USD), which can be a significant expense for practitioners worldwide. Third, EHB is a comprehensive resource with multiple features, allowing users to avoid downloading several different applications. It includes many different calculators (i.e. IOL calculators, glaucoma risk, etc.), patient assessment tools (amsler grid, visual acuity testing, OKN drum, etc.), medication information (indications, dosing, etc.),

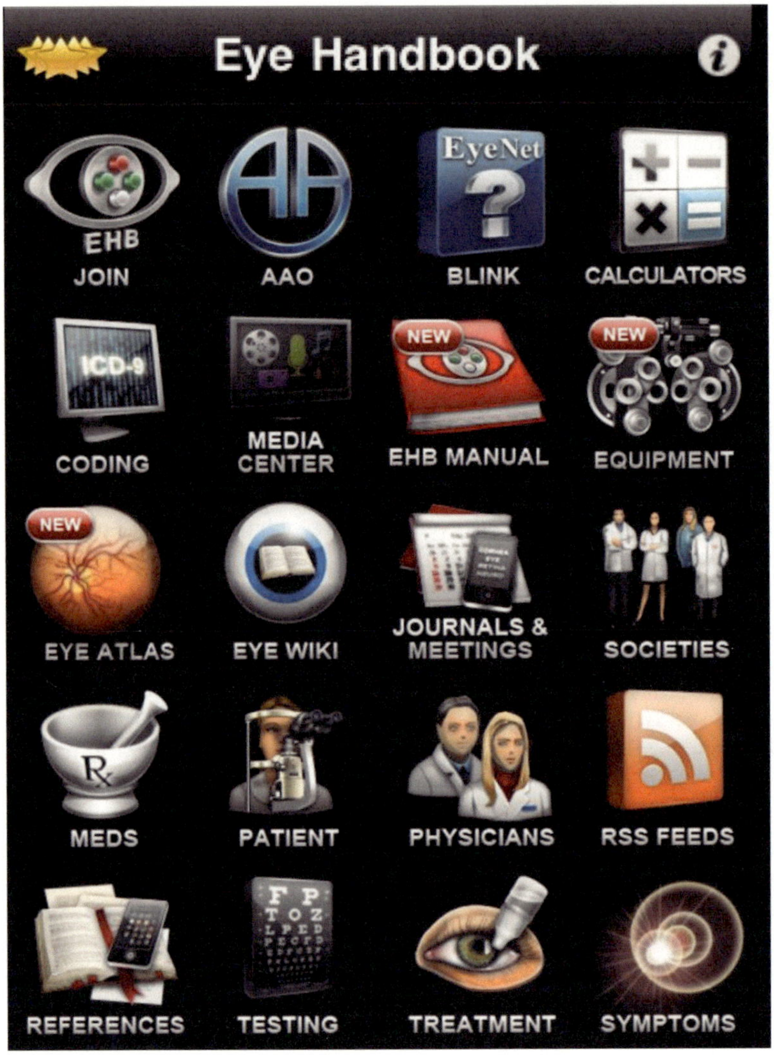

Figure 6.
Menu of The Eye Handbook smartphone application.

and much more. EHB also contains a comprehensive manual of different diseases and includes their epidemiology, pathophysiology, signs and symptoms, differential diagnosis, workup, treatment, and follow up – all of which can be incredibly useful for eye care professionals with limited ophthalmic training in LICs.

3.4 Smartphone-assisted fundoscopy

In addition to the scarcity of ophthalmologists globally, another challenge facing the fight against global blindness is the lack of ophthalmic equipment needed for proper eye care. Given the explosion of mobile phones that 96% of the world's population now owns, the innovations in fundus photography highlight the ability of smartphones to photograph the fundus [24] and use the smartphone in combination with a 20D condensing lens to capture wider field images of pathology [25].

Traditional ophthalmic equipment, such as office-based cameras are expensive, bulky, immobile and unsuitable for reaching patients in rural areas. Newer developments in technology are replacing our reliance on large equipment and allowing us to visualize the eye in a mobile and more cost-efficient manner. Smartphone-based technologies can now act as slit lamps, direct ophthalmoscopes, and indirect ophthalmoscopes. **Table 1** lists some of the products currently available. While these images will not be as sharp as those achieved with traditional cameras, they are of adequate resolution for interpretation. This development will allow eye care providers to have more access to imaging technologies, which provide imaging of harder-to-reach patients in rural areas with geo-tagging and wireless transfer of results to distantly-located specialists for appropriate management. One study found that even nonophthalmologists can be trained to effectively capture fundus images in a rural area [26]. This section draws greatly from the 2018 literature review by Barikian et al. [27].

Disadvantages of smartphone-based imaging are the high intensity of the phone light source, which constricts the pupil. However, applications such as Shutter can be used to tailor the intensity and exposure time of the flash for optimal illumination. Another disadvantage is achieving proper beam alignment.

In addition to smartphone-based imaging, standalone handheld camera technologies also allow portable image capture. These cameras are lightweight and capture quality retinal images. Examples of such devices include the Panoptic (Welch Allyn, Skaneateles Falls, NY), Volk Pictor (Volk Optical, Mentor, OH),

Category	Device	Manufacturer	Validated in LIC?	FoV	Pupillary dilation	Cost (USD)
Slit lamp imaging	EyePhotoDoc	EyePhotoDoc (Fullerton, CA)	No	N/A	Required	$300
	Portable Slit Lamp iPhone 4 Image Adapter	Keeler (Broomall, PA)	No	N/A	Required	$203
	SteadyPix Telescope Photoadapter	Orion (Cupertino, CA)	No	N/A	Required	$48
	Zarf iPhone Adapter	Zarf (Spokane, WA)	No	N/A	Required	$520
	Create-your-own adapter	www.instructables.com www.eyewiki.aao.org	No	N/A	Required	N/A
Direct ophthalmoscopy	iExaminer	Welch Allyn (Skaneateles Falls, NY)	No	25°	Optional	$800
	D-Eye Adapter	D-EYE (Padua, Italy)	No	20°	Optional	$435
	PEEK Retina	Peek Vision (London, UK)	Yes [28]	20–30°	Optional	$245
	Ocular Cellscope	University of California (Berkeley, CA)	No	55°	Required	N/A
	Remidio FOP	Remidio Innovative Solutions (Bangalore, India)	No	45°	Required	$6500
Indirect ophthalmoscopy	Smartphone and lens	Multiple	No	50°	Required	$200
	MII Ret Cam	MII Ret Cam (Coimbatore, India)	No	40–50°	Required	$350
	oDocs	Open source	No	40°	Required	$0
	Volk iNview	Volk Optical (Mentor, OH)	No	50°	Optional	$995

Table 1.
Products available for smartphone-based imaging.

VersaCam (Nidek, Gamagori, Japan), Horus Scope (JedMed, St. Louis, MO), and Smartscope (Optomed, Oulu, Finland). A limitation of such devices is the need for proper manual alignment of the illuminating beam with the optical axis for good-quality images. They also lack the ability to integrate with various apps as smartphone-based cameras and tend to be fragile. More importantly, these devices are cost-prohibitive for LICs.

3.5 Ultrasound

VuPad (Sonomed Escalon) and Accutome offer the only portable laptop size ultrasounds that can be used in low-income countries. They are expensive at over $10 k and do not yet accommodate smart phone utilization. Ultrasound (US) is a noninvasive, very easy to operate tool that plays an important role in clinical ophthalmology. It is used for the visualization of anatomy and various ocular pathology such as retinal detachment and intraocular tumors. Ultrasound becomes especially important if visualization of fundus becomes obscured by opaque elements including vitreous hemorrhage or dense mature cataracts commonly encountered in LIC. Butterfly iQ is the first portable US probe that can be plugged directly into a smartphone to visualize various parts of the body but is not yet approved for the eye (**Figure** 7). The probe uses a single silicone chip that replaces traditional transducer system. Clinicians can switch between various types of transducers, such as linear, curved or phased, without the need of switching probes. Moreover, the Butterfly iQ application allows clinicians to organize and remotely access imaging studies through the Butterfly Cloud. The Butterfly Cloud is HIPAA compliant and the application is developed in a way that makes it easy to share studies between various clinicians across the globe. Butterfly iQ weighs around 0.7 lbs. and is small enough to fit in pants pocket and costs about $2000. Butterfly iQ is being utilized for point of care ultrasound by physicians and emergency room physicians but could evolve as the first smartphone based ocular ultrasound. It has future potential to be used by visual care providers in resource poor areas for diagnosing ocular pathology.

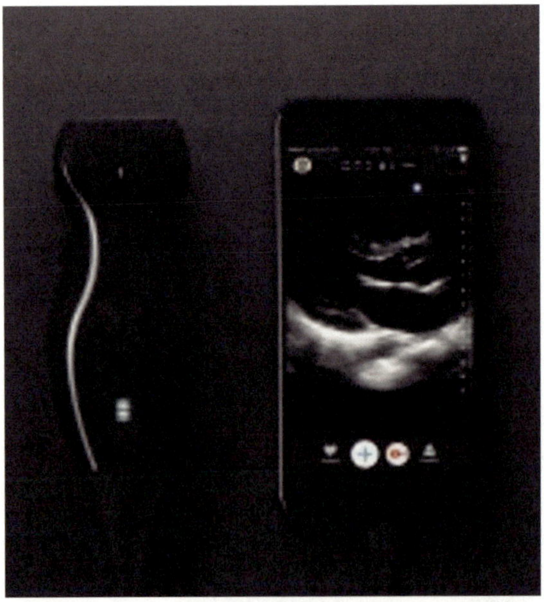

Figure 7.
Butterfly iQ is a portable ultrasound probe that can be plugged into any smartphone to visualize various anatomical features, including the eye.

The Clarus Portable Ultrasound is palm sized, connects to a wireless smartphone or tablet, but is not yet marketed for ophthalmology use. Its rugged, portable and waterproof design makes it ideal for global health (relief camp settings/medical missions) where it has been used for ophthalmology as part of a FAST exam.

A group from the University of Arizona assessed a new ultrasound system, the Vevo 2100 (VisualSonics, Toronto, Ontario, Canada) and its ability to examine structures of the anterior and posterior segments [28]. This system is unique in that it was able to implement high-frequency (>20 MHz) linear ultrasonic arrays that were not previously available in ophthalmic practice. Previous ultrasound technologies used single-element transducers, while the Vevo 2100 uses linear array technology with more than 100 piezoelectric elements packed into the face of the transducer probe. The new technology allows users to examine the eye quickly (approximately 10 seconds) with high resolution (30–60 μm). Additionally, it allows the scan to be shown in three-dimensions at different planes with sagittal, transverse, and coronal sections. This allows users to measure the location, dimensions, and volume of lesions or parts of the eye, which could be useful for providing information on the growth of lesions over time. The technology could also be used to determine the extent of traumatic injury and location of foreign bodies. A doppler function also allows examination of the temporal artery as well as vessels of the optic nerve head. However, despite the accurate images, the Vevo 2100 provides the anterior and posterior segments, and its high cost makes it a limiting factor for use in LIC.

3.6 mHealth in LICs

Mobile health, also referred to as mHealth, refers to the use of short messaging service (SMS), wireless data transfer, voice calling, and smartphone applications to transmit health-related information or direct medical care. A thorough 2013 systematic review by Betjeman et al. [29] found that mHealth can be a valuable tool in sub-Saharan Africa (SSA) to monitor patients, increase medication adherence, promote healthcare worker communication, and assist with disaster response. One of the key factors of mHealth is the prevalence of mobile phones even within LICs: penetration rates of mobile phones are greater than 70% in SSA [29].

mHealth has been shown to be a cost-effective means of improving medication adherence in LICs [29]. A study of 155 patients in South Africa tested the utility of SIMpill, a medication dispensing system that uses a SIM card to send an SMS text to a central server each time the medication bottle is opened (**Figure 8**). If the server does not receive an SMS before a preset time, a reminder text message is sent to the patient's mobile phone. If there is no response from the patient, an SMS is sent to the patient's healthcare provider for direct follow up. One study found that the SIMpill system increased medication adherence rates from 22–60 to 94% [30]. The WelTel Kenyal study found that even weekly SMS text messages inquiring about patient wellbeing is sufficient to increase self-reported medication adherence and HIV viral suppression [31]. The system deployed in this study cost under $8 USD per patient per year. Another study in Kenya used a combination of video messages and text messages, having the patient's friends or relatives capture video images of the patient taking their medication which is reviewed by nurses for follow up if there is low medication adherence. This study found that 50% of the messages were not received, mostly due to technical issues [32]. This demonstrates the need for a strong technological infrastructure in regions that mHealth is being deployed. Based on the results of these studies, mHealth can be an effective and cost-effective means to increase medication adherence in LICs with wireless network coverage.

mHealth can also be a means of increasing community health worker (CHW) access to health information, access to health information, decision making, and

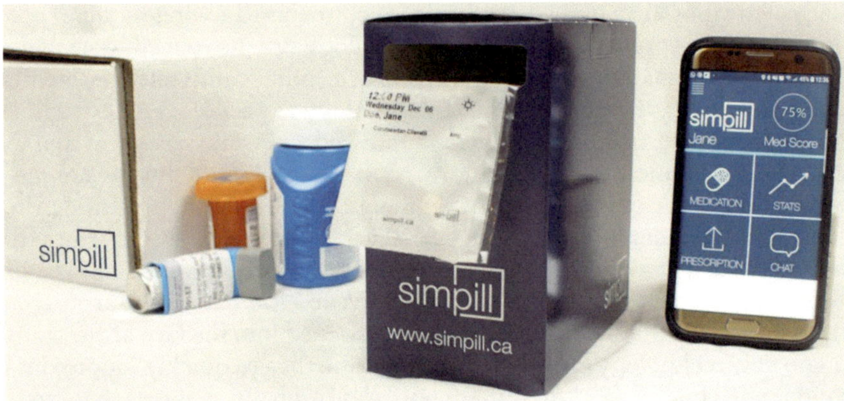

Figure 8.
The SIMpill system sends an SMS message to centrally-located servers, recording each time a patient takes their medication.

logistical support [29]. A study in Malawi found that CHWs most often used SMS to report supply shortages, communicate information with other CHW, and facilitate emergency communication [33]. Importantly, this study found that the average cost per communication using SMS was one-fifth the cost of communication in areas without SMS access. SMS communication took approximately 9 minutes, compared to 24 hours in areas without SMS access [33]. Another study found that common uses of SMS by CHW were patient referral, drug dosing information, emergency support, and reporting patient mortality. This study found that the efficiency of SMS communication substantially increased free time of hospital staff, allowing staff to treat more patients. These studies show that mHealth can significantly increase CHW efficiency while reducing overall healthcare costs in LICs.

mHealth could potentially be used to facilitate health education among patients in LICs [29]. One study sent an SMS squiz on HIV awareness to 10,000 cell phone subscribers and found significant challenges associated with the use of mHealth as a patient education tool [34]. First, the study found that individuals tended to only respond to questions for which they knew the correct answer, while skipping other questions. This demonstrates that it may be difficult to use mHealth to transmit new information to patients. Second, and perhaps more importantly, the study found that respondents were more likely to be men. The authors postulated this to be due to men having higher rates of mobile phone ownership and literacy. This could indicate future difficulty for mHealth to be used as an education tool for women in LICs.

3.7 Remote database access

Rapid Assessment of Avoidable Blindness (RAAB) is a survey system that estimates prevalence of avoidable blindness in a population over age 50. The data gathered from these surveys are stored in a repository, which not only details the prevalence of eye diseases and their causes but also the quality of eye services, resources and barriers to care in a specific geographical area. This resource is invaluable to researchers and country ministries of health, as it grants them easy access to data. Moreover, it allows agencies and eye care providers to focus their efforts on regions with the greatest medical need with optimal utilization of limited resources. These RAAB surveys can also be completed using a smartphone application developed by the PEEK Vision project called mRAAB [35]. The mRAAB application has increased the quality and efficiency of data entry by allowing the data to be entered while the examiner is still with the patient. It has been tested successfully in countries such as Tanzania, the Maldives, Madagascar, Uganda, Zimbabwe, and Nigeria. The future goal of mRAAB is to integrate PEEK functions such as visual acuity assessments and ocular photography with the surveys.

The Open Data Kit is another mobile data collection application that has facilitated the collection, management, and access to data in remote and resource-limited regions. It is a free and open-source software that is already being used by organizations such as the WHO, Red Cross, and Red Crescent [36]. Similar to the mRAAB, this is a great resource that allows various eye care organizations and providers to collect and share data that can increase the effectiveness of their efforts.

Poor cataract outcomes are often detected in RAAB surveys of cataract patients in sub-Saharan Africa. The WHO recommends Better Operative Outcomes Software Technology (BOOST) to track cataract surgery cases for quality assessment and improvement. BOOST is an application developed by several nongovernmental organizations and the Aravind Eye Hospital (Madurai, India) which allows cataract surgeons to measure and benchmark their surgical results against others in a cloud-based database. It also provides advice on how to improve outcomes [37]. The app uses two rounds of data collection. First, users measure visual acuity of patients the day after surgery to measure the proportion of patients with good (defined as >6/18) and bad (defined as <6/60) visual acuity. Second, for patients returning 6 weeks postoperatively with vision less than 6/60, users choose from among three reasons for poor vision outcomes (refractive problems, surgical misadventure, presence of ocular comorbidity). The app then suggests changes in practice for users to help improve their most common causes of poor vision.

3.8 Simulations in cataract surgery

Simulation-based training for cataract surgery is an innovation with substantial promise for treating global blindness in LIC. Cataracts account for nearly half of all cases of global blindness, the majority being in the developing world [38]. While many of these cases can be cured with inexpensive surgical procedures, there is a shortage of surgeons to handle the caseload. Trainees in developing countries face a lack of equipment and teaching personnel. Simulation-based training could help alleviate this shortage of surgeons by providing practice cases without the requirement for actual patients. Several simulators currently exist on the market, including HelpMeSee (HelpMeSee, New York), Eyesi (VRmagic, Manheim, Germany), MicroVisTouch (ImmersiveTouch, Chicago), and Phacovision (Melerit Medical, Linköping, Sweden), among others.

The Eyesi is the most prevalent of commercially available simulators in U.S. and European ophthalmology residency programs [39]. It is a high-fidelity phacoemulsification simulator. The hardware consists of a mannequin headpiece with a mechanical eye, which is wired to a computer interface and a microscope, allowing the trainee to assume the most realistic posture (**Figure 9**). Eyesi also includes surgical instruments and foot pedals. The system allows users to watch previous surgeries to review and improve upon. It consists of different learning modules, including anti-tremor training, bimanual training, capsulorhexis, cracking and chopping training, forceps training, hydro-dissection maneuvers, intraocular lens insertion, irrigation and aspiration, navigation training, and phacoemulsification training. VRmagic also produces Eyesi indirect and direct ophthalmoscopes for simulation-based training in ophthalmoscopy (**Figures 10** and **11**). The HMS system includes a platform similar to the Eyesi system with a microscope, monitor, and instruments attached to robotic arms (**Figure 12**). The MicroVisTouch system includes a blunt-tip handpiece attached to a robotic arm, with a mannequin headpiece to practice proper hand placement. The handpiece serves as the appropriate

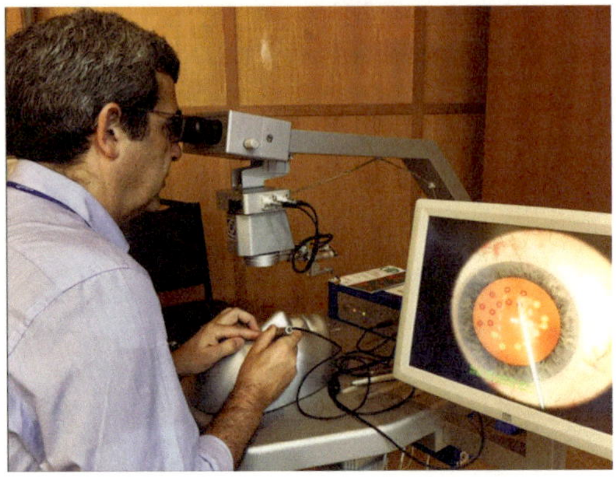

Figure 9.
The VRmagic Eyesi surgical simulator allows users to go through modules of high fidelity simulations of phacoemulsification and vitreoretinal surgery steps.

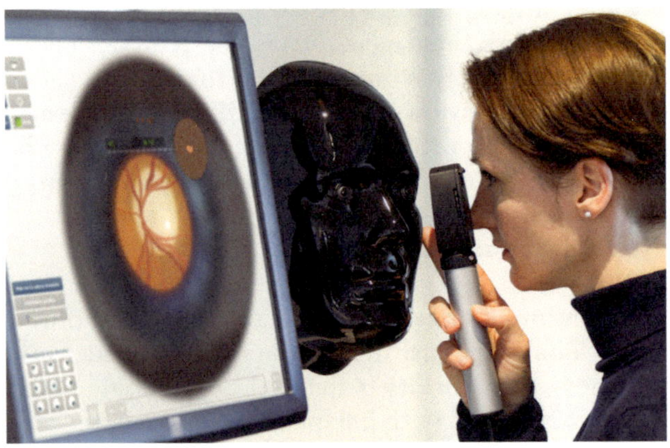

Figure 10.
The VRmagic direct ophthalmoscope allows users to develop the skillset for direct ophthalmoscopy by progressively moving through skill modules and case pathology.

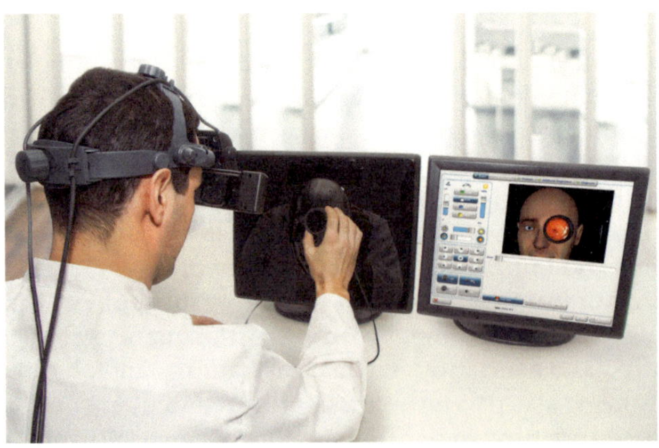

Figure 11.
The VRmagic indirect ophthalmoscope allows users to develop the skillset for binocular indirect ophthalmoscopy with a 20D and 28D lens and records the percentage of the retina visualized in focus by the examiner.

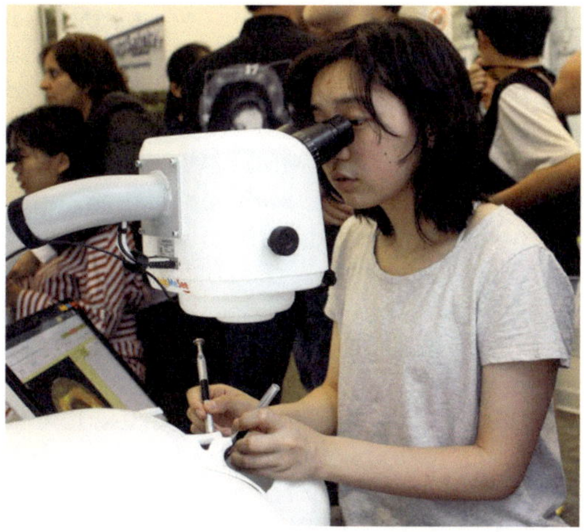

Figure 12.
The HelpMeSee simulation system allows users to practice small incision cataract surgery (SICS).

instrument based on the stage of surgery being performed, from a keratome to forceps. The system also includes haptic feedback, a relatively new addition to the market for surgery simulators.

A 2015 systematic review of by Thomsen et al. found the overall evidence of research in the use of simulators as both training and assessment tools to be inadequate [40]. Another recent study by Thomsen [41] tested the Eyesi as a training method of 18 surgeons of varying levels of experience. Each surgeon was graded based on a previously-validated testing tool for cataract surgery (Objective Structured Assessment of Cataract Surgical Skill). The study found that novice surgeons benefited by training on the Eyesi, while more experienced surgeons did not. Compared with no intervention, simulation-based training has been shown to have large improvements in user knowledge, skills, and behaviors, along with moderate improvements in patient outcomes across many surgical and medical fields [42]. Given the lack of training institutions, wet labs, etc., in LICs, the use of simulators can play a key role in training future cataract surgeons.

3.9 The HelpMeSee approach to cataract-induced blindness

A 2013 review by Broyles et al. explains that HMS is doing more than simply creating cataract simulation technology. Despite the aforementioned shortcomings in the research of simulators, the organization is creating training centers around the world that incorporate surgical simulation as well as traditional learning methods, centered around a textbook written at an 8th grade English level. Their goal is to fight global blindness caused by cataracts. These training centers will be located within LICs such as Asia, Africa, and Latin America. The intended trainee will include health care professionals and individuals without medical training in order to create the manpower necessary to meet the global need for surgeons. However, HMS predicts that 60% of the trainees will be physicians. Each center will have the capacity to train approximately 1000 trainees per year. Only those who successfully complete the cognitive training will move forward to surgical training, where they will be trained in manual small incision cataract surgery (MSICS), a safe, low-cost, and rapid method for surgical cataract removal compared to other costlier methods.

The graduates then become part of a network of independently-functioning MSICS practitioners that are responsible for seeking out treatable cataract cases in their practicing area, providing surgical care on a fee-for-service basis, and reporting quality metrics via electronic photographs to HMS. The practitioners will live and work in the underserved areas HMS hopes to serve. By focusing only on cataract surgery, the intention is to create high surgical volumes per practitioner in order to drive unit costs of surgery sufficiently low and maintain surgeons' skills. Depending on uptake of surgical services, the cost per surgery could be as low as $69 in southeast Asia. Better skill and outcomes will then drive local credibility and encourage uptake of the program by locals.

The review forecast that the HMS is able to train 30,000 new surgeons. It also models different levels of uptake of HMS surgeries: low (20% of cataract-caused visually impaired individuals not operated on elsewhere are operated on by HMS), medium (50% operated on by HMS), and high (80% operated on by HMS). With these assumptions, the model predicts that the projected 134 million individuals with cataract-caused blindness in the four identified regions can be reduced to 21 million individuals in the case of high uptake (80%). The reductions are more modest in the medium and low uptake assumptions. The economic effect, with visually-impaired individuals now able to work, would mean an additional $52 billion of GDP in the Western Pacific Region (i.e., China) if the high scenario is met. The increase in GDP would be $18 billion in Southeast Asia and $9 billion in the Africa region. However, once the cataract surgery backlog is eliminated, there will likely be an oversupply of surgeons. The timeframe depends on the uptake of surgical services by region but could be as soon as 2021 in the African region. After that point, surgeons would rely on new cases of cataracts for business. Surgeons could then possibly serve as referral sources for broader ophthalmic services to larger care organizations.

The HMS system faces several obstacles. First, training a new cohort of high-quality cataract surgeons in an efficient manner will likely pose many challenges. Second, it may be challenging for local practitioners to educate patients on the need for surgery and bring in sufficient volumes of cases to drive the unit cost sufficiently low. It will also be difficult for surgeons to have the high surgical load and make time for patient screening and outreach. Third, it may be difficult for individuals to travel the distance required to have the surgery. While the surgeons will live in the regions they serve; patients living in rural will likely still need to travel significant distances for care. This challenge could be reduced by providing transportation services at the time of screening by other qualified medical staff. Fourth, patients with non-cataract pathologies could be disappointed by the inability of practitioners to treat their disease. This could discourage local credibility and would require the practitioner to market their services appropriately. Fifth, it will be challenging for HMS to monitor quality of care provided due to the volume of surgeons operating in multiple different regions worldwide. This increases the need for technology-driven quality monitoring via sophisticated imaging.

4. International organizations promoting visual health

There are several leading global organizations dedicated to providing vision care. Vision Springs, Eyelliance, Eyesee and Vision for a Nation are some of the organizations that focus on providing eyeglasses to low-income countries. Vision Springs is an organization that relies on a high-volume low margin business model. It employs optical shops in communities with limited access to eye care services. These optical shops provide eye exams and low-cost prescription glasses to the community. Vision Springs also partners with local NGOs and businesses to distribute eyeglasses using their already established distribution channels. This model allows them to distribute glasses to areas in need while keeping the cost as low as possible. Eyelliance and Vision for a Nation follow a similar model. Eyesee is a student-run organization based in the U.S which collects used eyeglasses and distribute them to the poor regions. Since its establishment in 2008, the organization has delivered free recycled glasses to countries such as Haiti, Nigeria, Uganda, Honduras, and Cambodia.

Another leading organization in global vision care is ORBIS. It is a non-profit organization based in New York that operates the Flying Eye Hospital. This mobile hospital is the only one of its kind in the world that provides eye restoration interventions in addition to education and training of local ophthalmic communities throughout low-income countries. The organization has been successful in establishing educational programs in countries such as Bangladesh, Ethiopia, India, and Vietnam. These programs have since provided treatments and prevention of various ocular diseases like cataracts and trachoma to their communities. ORBIS also launched a telemedicine initiative in 2003 called Cybersight. Through Cybersight, ophthalmologists in the U.S. are able to connect 24/7 with local community physicians worldwide to offer them with professional consultation and education on various surgical techniques and patient cases.

The International Agency for the Prevention of Blindness (IAPB), established in 1975, is one of the major organizations that leads international endeavors toward blindness intervention. Through its efforts, Vision 2020 was able to be formed in collaboration with the WHO. The organization's goal in the years between 2013 and 2017 was to promote access to eye health particularly in the most marginalized regions of the world. As a result, IAPB sponsors variety of global initiatives such as Seeing is Believing, the DR Barometer Project, Our Children's Vision, The Rotary International Service Partnership, and the Vision Alliance [43].

5. Future prospects

One of the most exciting emerging frontiers in ophthalmology is the ability of automated devices to diagnose and treat various ocular diseases through artificial intelligence (AI). Giant technology companies such as Google and IBM have dedicated plenty of resources to developing their own version of AI systems. Such systems have shown great promise in playing an important role in patient care. For example, Google Brain (AI system developed by Google) was able to detect the spread of breast cancer by examining microscopic specimen images of lymph nodes. In fact, Google Brain's performance was comparable and, in some cases, superior to that of human pathologists [44]. Similar developments are occurring in ophthalmology, in particularly the field of retinal diseases. In 2016, Google Brian's AI system through machine learning was able to "learn" how detect diabetic retinopathy and diabetic macular edema from funduscopic photographs [45]. New systems are currently being developed to evaluate other ophthalmic disorders such as cataract, glaucoma and keratoconus.

These intelligent systems could prove invaluable in global health with the potential to improve health care affordability, efficiency and accessibility. The system can act as an adjunct for eye care capacity building. For example, it could enable non-medical personnel with a few hours of training to diagnose ocular disease without physicians' interpretation, in turn, expanding medical care to remote regions without practicing ophthalmologists. In addition to serving as a solution to the increased shortage of ophthalmologists in low-income countries through simplifying the process of diagnosing ocular diseases, ocular pathology can be diagnosed at earlier stages. Diagnosing diseases at earlier stages will allow for earlier intervention and in turn yielding better medical outcomes. Moreover, with identification of populations with greater disease burden, resources can be focused on those areas for treatment to maximize its utility.

The US Food and Drug Administration has recently made history by approving the first AI retinal diagnostic system called IDx-DR. The system specializes in autonomously detecting diabetic retinopathy, one of the major causes of vision loss and blindness worldwide. For example, in India, the WHO estimates that around 32 million people were affected by diabetes mellitus (DM) in 2000. We expect the epidemiologic curve to shift from infectious, communicable diseases to non-communicable diseases in the next decade. By 2030, in India alone, these figures are expected to increase to around 80 million people vulnerable to developing diabetic retinopathy [46]. Vision loss, as result of this disease, can be easily controlled with early detection and management; however, most patients with diabetes in low-income countries end up without any eye care. However, IDx-DR currently is only validated and approved by the FDA for use in the US.

IDx-DR could be a future health solution to identify patients with greatest risk early in the disease process, in turn maximizing limited physician resources by focusing on patients who need advanced care. Using a fundus camera, an operator, who does not require previous ophthalmology knowledge, captures two images per eye (**Figure 13**). These images are automatically sent to a computer system that analyzes the images for any signs of diabetic retinopathy. In less than a minute the computer stratifies eyes into two groups. Group 1 contains eyes that are negative or demonstrate mild diabetic retinopathy while Group 2 contains eyes with stages more advanced than mild diabetic retinopathy. Group 1 can be retested in 12 months while group 2 is referred to an eye care specialist. A recent study demonstrated IDx-DR to have similar sensitivity in detecting diabetic retinopathy to human experts [47].

With future system improvement, the integration of this intelligent screening system in a portable fundus camera or a smartphone will greatly improve its accessibility to remote regions. Moreover, having the ability to diagnose diabetic retinopathy (and other ocular diseases in the future) in a matter of few seconds will provide the efficiency to screen larger populations. This new emerging AI technology is a major breakthrough in global health and will serve to positively impact the visual health of millions of patients.

Another major cause of visual impairment worldwide is uncorrected refractive error. In fact, it is considered to be the leading cause of visual impairment worldwide, as more than 650 million people suffer from lack of adequate refractive error

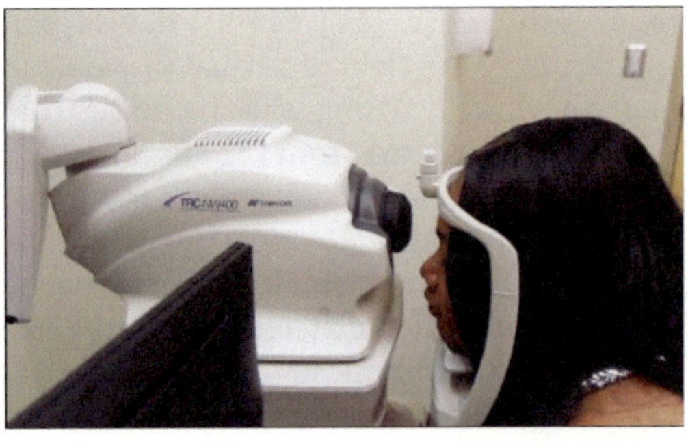

Figure 13.
IDx-DR uses artificial intelligence to detect diabetic retinopathy without the need for experienced ophthalmologic personnel.

correction [48, 49]. It is estimated that the resulting visual impairment contributes to more than 250 billion dollars in productivity loss [48]. This loss of income can be very detrimental, especially to low-income countries where individuals make less than one dollar a day. Providing adequate vision screening and refractive error correction can be very cost effective. A study called PROductivity Study of Presbyopia Elimination in Rural-dwellers (PROSPER), was published in 2018 showed a clear link between refractive error correction and productivity increase [50]. The study conducted in India looked at tea pickers with uncorrected refractive error. It found that providing workers with corrective lenses improved their productivity by 21.7%. Therefore, providing adequate screening and eyeglasses offers an easy solution for the reversal of low vision and blindness, leading to improved quality of life and economic development worldwide. In fact, the WHO considers refractive error as one of the priority eye diseases that it aims to combat globally.

Phoropter is the most widely used tools by ophthalmologists and optometrists to measure patients' refractive error and determine the eyeglass prescription strength. It relies on a heavy set of numerous spherical and cylindrical lenses of various powers. A large number of lenses is required for examination since, eyecare providers must cover the refractive error conditions such as myopia, hyperopia, and astigmatism, along with their respective degree of impairment. This can make mobility of eye care personnel and transportation of equipment between sites a burdensome task, especially in remote areas where road systems are underdeveloped. Moreover, the process of finding the proper prescription strength requires constant patient feedback in order to determine the lens power that provides the sharpest image. It is a very time-consuming process that can limit the number of patients seen by an eye specialist. Moreover, the communication element can be very challenging in certain populations such as children and elderly or patients with mental disabilities or cognitive impairments. It also requires either the eyecare providers speak the language of their patients or the availability of an interpreter in order for the test to be completed. This can force providers to avoid regions where language is a barrier.

A solution to the aforementioned limitations is currently being developed by a team from Tucson, Arizona called the auto-phoropter [51]. The auto-phoropter is a low-cost handheld device that is able to measure a patient's refractive without the need of patient's feedback. In contrast to the already available autorefractors, the auto-phoropter does not require fine tuning of patient's refractive error measurement with an additional exam using lens trials. The special system of lenses and sensors in the auto-phoropter make measuring the refractive error possible. The device contains three separate fluidic lenses, two cylindrical lenses that are placed 45° with respect to each other for astigmatism correction and a spherical lens for myopia/hyperopia. Through pressure induced deformation by the liquid that is pumped in and out of the lens, the power of the fluidic lens can be tuned in increments of 0.1 diopters. With a special wavefront sensor which measures the infrared wavefront coming from the eye called Shack-Hartmann, the refractive error can be calculated in matter of seconds. As a result, the device portability, lack of patient's subjective feedback and the prompt corrective error measurement, the auto-phoropter will allow large patient population screening without the need of trained eye specialists.

According to one estimate, there are more than 1 billion people above the age of 35 that are suffering from uncorrected presbyopia while more than 200 million people suffer from moderate and severe vision impairment (<6/18 but better than 3/60) [52]. Giving patients eyeglasses after vision testing will ensure that they receive the appropriate intervention instead of solely providing them with a prescription. There are various of factors that might impair patients from following up and getting their custom-made glasses. These factors include cost and lack of perceived benefit to name a few. Therefore, as expected, it will be much more likely that patients wear eyeglasses if offered for free, rather than for purchase [50]. For this reason, we recommend that screening programs carry both reading and prescription glasses to cover the whole spectrum of refraction errors, especially in areas that lack the appropriate facilities and resources.

Nevertheless, being able to carry large number of glasses can be challenging both logistically and financially. Ordering eyeglasses in bulk will help lower their individual cost. We found that in some factories in China, manufacturing a pair of reading glasses can cost as little as USD 0.50 while a prescription glasses for myopia can cost around USD 1.50. Adjustable glasses can be a solution to reducing the number of eyeglass carried by screening programs. However, this advanced type of eyeglasses is more expensive, as a pair can cost around USD 19.

6. Conclusion

This chapter outlined various emerging diagnostic tools and resources that aim to assist in the fight against preventable blindness and achieve the mission of Vision 2020. From Web-based databases and global organizations to smartphone applications and diagnostic devices, eye care providers have emerging diagnostic tools to promote visual health and increase access in global underserved areas. We hope that with the continual evolution of technology, and with improved accessibility and affordability of visual care, preventable blindness can be 1 day eliminated worldwide.

Acknowledgements

The authors would like to thank the Global Retina Institute, Scottsdale, Arizona (USA) for research funding and special thanks to VRmagic (Mannheim, Germany) and Peek Vision Ltd. (England) for use of images.

Conflict of interest

The authors have no conflict of interest.

DOI: http://dx.doi.org/10.5772/intechopen.83455

Author details

Jason Singh[1], Sami Kabbara[1], Mandi Conway[1], Gholam Peyman[1] and Robin D. Ross[2,3]*

1 Department of Ophthalmology, University of Arizona College of Medicine—Phoenix, United States

2 Department of Bioethics and Medical Humanism, Phoenix, Arizona, United States

3 Global Retina Institute, Scottsdale, Arizona, United States

*Address all correspondence to: rross@globalretinainstitute.com

References

[1] Fricke TR, Tahhan N, Resnikoff S, et al. Global prevalence of presbyopia and vision impairment from uncorrected presbyopia: Systematic review, meta-analysis, and modelling. Ophthalmology. 2018;**125**(10):1492-1499

[2] Bourne RR, Stevens GA, White RA, et al. Causes of vision loss worldwide, 1990-2010: A systematic analysis. The Lancet Global Health. 2013;**1**(6):e339-e349

[3] World Health Organization. Blindness and Vision Impairment Prevention. Available from: http://www.who.int/blindness/causes/priority/en/index3.html [Accessed: Oct 24, 2018]

[4] Pizzarello L, Abiose A, Ffytche T, et al. VISION 2020: The right to sight: A global initiative to eliminate avoidable blindness. Archives of Ophthalmology. 2004;**122**(4):615-620

[5] Palmer JJ, Chinanayi F, Gilbert A, et al. Mapping human resources for eye health in 21 countries of sub-Saharan Africa: Current progress towards VISION 2020. Human Resources for Health. 2014;**12**:44. DOI: 10.1186/1478-4491-12-44

[6] Naidoo KS, Leasher J, Bourne RR, et al. Global vision impairment and blindness due to uncorrected refractive error, 1990-2010. Optometry and Vision Science. 2016;**93**(3):227-234

[7] Dandona R, Dandona L, Kovai V, Giridhar P, Prasad MN, Srinivas M. Population-based study of spectacles use in southern India. Indian Journal of Ophthalmology. 2002;**50**(2):145-155

[8] Mathenge W, Nkurikiye J, Limburg H, Kuper H. Rapid assessment of avoidable blindness in western Rwanda: Blindness in a postconflict setting. PLoS Medicine. 2007;**4**(7):e217

[9] Number of eye care professionals in the United States in 2014 and 2020 (in 1,000). 2016. Available from: http://www.statista.com/statistics/448742/eye-care-professionals-in-the-us-Forecast/

[10] Bastawrous A, Rono HK, Livingstone IA, et al. Development and validation of a smartphone-based visual acuity test (Peek Acuity) for clinical practice and community-based fieldwork. JAMA Ophthalmology. 2015;**133**(8):930-937

[11] Lodhia V, Karanja S, Lees S, Bastawrous A. Acceptability, usability, and views on deployment of peek, a mobile phone mHealth intervention for eye care in Kenya: Qualitative study. JMIR mHealth uHealth. 2016;**4**(2):e30

[12] Rono HK, Bastawrous A, Macleod D, et al. Smartphone-based screening for visual impairment in Kenyan school children: A cluster randomised controlled trial. The Lancet Global Health. 2018;**6**(8):e924-e932

[13] Optical Society of America. NETRA-G: Towards a Subjective Self-Refraction. 2014. Available from: https://eyenetra.com/studies/Frontiers%20In%20Optics%20-%20NETRA.pdf [Accessed: Oct 20, 2018]

[14] Arnold RW, O'Neil JW, Cooper KL, Silbert DI, Donahue SP. Evaluation of a smartphone photoscreening app to detect refractive amblyopia risk factors in children aged 1-6 years. Clinical Ophthalmology. 2018;**12**:1533-1537. [Published Aug 23, 2018]. DOI: 10.2147/OPTH.S171935

[15] Whiteman H. Self-adjustable eyeglasses: How one man's vision is helping others to see better. Medical News Today. 2015. Available from: https://www.medicalnewstoday.com/articles/302550.php [Accessed: Oct 24, 2018]

[16] Camp AS, Shane TS, Kang J, Thomas B, Pole C, Lee RK. Evaluating self-refraction and ready-made spectacles for treatment of uncorrected refractive error. Ophthalmic Epidemiology. 2018;**25**(5-6):392-398

[17] Zhang M, Zhang R, He M, et al. Self correction of refractive error among young people in rural China: Results of cross sectional investigation. British Medical Journal. 2011;**343**:d4767

[18] He M, Congdon N, MacKenzie G, Zeng Y, Silver JD, Ellwein L. The child self-refraction study results from urban Chinese children in Guangzhou. Ophthalmology. 2011;**118**(6):1162-1169

[19] Annadanam A, Varadaraj V, Mudie LI, et al. Comparison of self-refraction using a simple device, USee, with manifest refraction in adults. PLoS One. 2018;**13**(2):e0192055

[20] Ramke J, du Toit R, Palagyi A, Brian G, Naduvilath T. Correction of refractive error and presbyopia in Timor-Leste. The British Journal of Ophthalmology. 2007;**91**(7):860-866

[21] Bastawrous A, Cheeseman RC, Kumar A. iPhones for eye surgeons. Eye (London, England). 2012;**26**(3):343-354

[22] Lord K, Shah VA, Krishna R. The eye handbook: A mobile app in ophthalmic medicine. Missouri Medicine. 2013;**110**(1):49-51

[23] Chhablani J, Kaja S, Shah VA. Smartphones in ophthalmology. Indian Journal of Ophthalmology. 2012;**60**(2):127-131

[24] Lord RK, Shah VA, San-Filippo AN, Krishna R. Novel uses of smartphones in ophthalmology. Ophthalmology. 2010;**117**(6):1274-1274.e3. DOI: 10.1016/j.ophtha.2010.01.001

[25] Shanmugam MP, Mishra DK, Madhukumar R, Ramanjulu R, Reddy SY, Rodrigues G. Fundus imaging with a mobile phone: A review of techniques. Indian Journal of Ophthalmology. 2014;**62**(9):960-962. DOI: 10.4103/0301-4738.143949

[26] Russo A, Morescalchi F, Costagliola C, Delcassi L, Semeraro F. Comparison of smartphone ophthalmoscopy with slit-lamp biomicroscopy for grading diabetic retinopathy. American Journal of Ophthalmology. 2015;**159**(2): 360-364, e1

[27] Barikian A, Haddock LJ. Smartphone assisted fundus fundoscopy/photography. Current Ophthalmology Reports. 2018;**6**:46-52. DOI: 10.1007/s40135-018-0162-7

[28] Peyman GA, Ingram CP, Montilla LG, Witte RS. A high-resolution 3D ultrasonic system for rapid evaluation of the anterior and posterior segment. Ophthalmic Surgery, Lasers & Imaging. 2012;**43**(2):143-151

[29] Betjeman TJ, Soghoian SE, Foran MP. mHealth in Sub-Saharan Africa. International Journal of Telemedicine and Applications. 2013;**2013**:482324

[30] Barclay E. Text messages could hasten tuberculosis drug compliance. The Lancet. 2009;**373**(9657):15-16

[31] Lester RT, Ritvo P, Mills EJ, et al. Effects of a mobile phone short message service on antiretroviral treatment adherence in Kenya (WelTel Kenya1): A randomised trial. The Lancet. 2010;**376**(9755):1838-1845

[32] Mahmud N, Rodriguez J, Nesbit J. A text message-based intervention to bridge the healthcare communication gap in the rural developing world. Technology and Health Care. 2010;**18**(2):137-144

[33] Lemay NV, Sullivan T, Jumbe B, Perry CP. Reaching remote health workers in Malawi: Baseline assessment

of a pilot mHealth intervention. Journal of Health Communication. 2012;**17**(supplement 1):105-117

[34] Chib A, Wilkin H, Ling LX, Hoefman B, van Biejma H. You have an important message! Evaluating the effectiveness of a text message HIV/AIDS campaign in Northwest Uganda. Journal of Health Communication. 2012;**17**(supplement 1):146-157

[35] RAAB Repository. mRAAB and PEEK. Available from: http://raabdata.info/about-the-raab-repository/mraab-and-peek/ [Accessed: Oct 24, 2018]

[36] International Federation of Red Cross and Red Crescent Societies. Bolivian Red Cross and IFRC Visit Border between Bolivia and Brazil. 2016. Available from: http://www.ifrc.org/en/news-and-media/news-stories/americas/bolivia/bolivian-red-cross-and-ifrc-visits-border-between-bolivia-and-brazil--72334/ [Accessed: Oct 24, 2018]

[37] Congdon N. Transforming research results into useful tools for global health: BOOST. The Lancet Website. 2016. Available from: https://www.thelancet.com/journals/langlo/article/PIIS2214-109X(15)00267-3/fulltext [Accessed: Oct 24, 2018]

[38] Broyles JR, Glick P, Hu J, Lim YW. Cataract blindness and simulation-based training for cataract surgeons: An assessment of the HelpMeSee approach. Rand Health Quarterly. 2013;**3**(1):7

[39] Brennan K. Imitation of life: Phaco simulators. Review of Ophthalmology Website. Available from: https://www.reviewofophthalmology.com/article/imitation-of-life-phaco-simulators. 2017. [Accessed: Oct 24, 2018]

[40] Thomsen AS, Subhi Y, Kiilgaard JF, la Cour M, Konge L. Update on simulation-based surgical training and assessment in ophthalmology: A systematic review. Ophthalmology. 2015;**122**(6):1111-1130, e1

[41] Thomsen ASS et al. Operating room performance improves after proficiency-based virtual reality cataract surgery training. Ophthalmology. 2017;**124**(4):524-531

[42] Cook DA, Hatala R, Brydges R, et al. Technology-enhanced simulation for health professions education: A systematic review and meta-analysis. JAMA 2011;**306**:978-988

[43] The International Agency for the Prevention of Blindness. Available from: https://www.iapb.org [Accessed: Oct 24, 2018]

[44] Cornell University Library. Detecting Cancer metastases on gigapixel pathology images. Available from: https://arxiv.org/pdf/1703.02442.pdf [Accessed: Oct 19, 2018]

[45] Srinivasan S, Shetty S, Natarajan V, Sharma T, Raman R. Development and validation of a diabetic retinopathy referral algorithm based on single-field fundus photography. PLoS One. 2016;**11**(9):e0163108

[46] Wild S, Roglic G, Green A, Sicree R, King H. Global prevalence of diabetes: Estimates for the year 2000 and projections for 2030. Diabetes Care. 2004;**27**:1047-1053

[47] van der Heijden AA, Abramoff MD, Verbraak F, van Hecke MV, Liem A, Nijpels G. Validation of automated screening for referable diabetic retinopathy with the IDx-DR device in the Hoorn diabetes care system. Acta Ophthalmologica. 2017;**96**(1):63-68

[48] Pascolini D, Mariotti SP. Global estimates of visual impairment: 2010. The British Journal of Ophthalmology. 2012;**96**(5):614-618

[49] Global, regional, and national incidence, prevalence, and years lived with disability for 301 acute and chronic diseases and injuries in 188 countries, 1990-2013: A systematic analysis for the global burden of disease study 2013. Lancet. 2015;**386**(9995):743-800

[50] Reddy PA, Congdon N, MacKenzie G, et al. Effect of providing near glasses on productivity among rural Indian tea workers with presbyopia (PROSPER): A randomised trial. The Lancet Global Health. 2018;**6**(9):e1019-e1027

[51] Amirsolaimani B, Peyman G, Schwiegerling J, Bablumyan A, Peyghambarian N. A new low-cost, compact, auto-phoropter for refractive assessment in developing countries. Scientific Reports 2017;7(1):13990 [Published Oct 25, 2017]. DOI: 10.1038/s41598-017-14507-5

[52] Bourne RRA, Flaxman SR, Braithwaite T, et al. Magnitude, temporal trends, and projections of the global prevalence of blindness and distance and near vision impairment: A systematic review and meta-analysis. The Lancet Global Health. 2017;**5**(9):e888-e897